Searching Skills Toolkit

17.99

Commissioning Editor: Mary Banks
Development Editor: Laura Beaumont

Searching Skills Toolkit

Finding the Evidence

by

Caroline De Brún
Librarian
National Library for Health
Oxford, UK

Nicola Pearce-Smith
Information Scientist
Department of Knowledge and Information Science
Summertown Pavilion
Middle Way
Oxford, UK

edited by

Carl Heneghan
Clinical Research Fellow
Department of Primary Health Care
University of Oxford
Oxford, UK

Rafael Perera
Centre for Evidence-based Medicine
Department of Primary Health Care
University of Oxford
Oxford, UK

Douglas Badenoch
Minervation Ltd
Oxford, UK

WILEY-BLACKWELL   BMJ|Books

This edition first published 2009, © 2009 by Caroline De Brún and Nicola Pearce-Smith

BMJ Books is an imprint of BMJ Publishing Group Limited, used under licence by Blackwell Publishing which was acquired by John Wiley & Sons in February 2007. Blackwell's publishing programme has been merged with Wiley's global Scientific, Technical and Medical business to form Wiley-Blackwell.

Registered office: John Wiley & Sons Ltd, The Atrium, Southern Gate, Chichester, West Sussex, PO19 8SQ, UK

Editorial offices: 9600 Garsington Road, Oxford, OX4 2DQ, UK
                       The Atrium, Southern Gate, Chichester, West Sussex, PO19 8SQ, UK
                       111 River Street, Hoboken, NJ 07030-5774, USA

For details of our global editorial offices, for customer services and for information about how to apply for permission to reuse the copyright material in this book please see our website at www.wiley.com/wiley-blackwell

The right of the author to be identified as the author of this work has been asserted in accordance with the Copyright, Designs and Patents Act 1988.

Wiley also publishes its books in a variety of electronic formats. Some content that appears in print may not be available in electronic books.

Designations used by companies to distinguish their products are often claimed as trademarks. All brand names and product names used in this book are trade names, service marks, trademarks or registered trademarks of their respective owners. The publisher is not associated with any product or vendor mentioned in this book. This publication is designed to provide accurate and authoritative information in regard to the subject matter covered. It is sold on the understanding that the publisher is not engaged in rendering professional services. If professional advice or other expert assistance is required, the services of a competent professional should be sought.

The contents of this work are intended to further general scientific research, understanding, and discussion only and are not intended and should not be relied upon as recommending or promoting a specific method, diagnosis, or treatment by physicians for any particular patient. The publisher and the author make no representations or warranties with respect to the accuracy or completeness of the contents of this work and specifically disclaim all warranties, including without limitation any implied warranties of fitness for a particular purpose. In view of ongoing research, equipment modifications, changes in governmental regulations, and the constant flow of information relating to the use of medicines, equipment, and devices, the reader is urged to review and evaluate the information provided in the package insert or instructions for each medicine, equipment, or device for, among other things, any changes in the instructions or indication of usage and for added warnings and precautions. Readers should consult with a specialist where appropriate. The fact that an organization or Website is referred to in this work as a citation and/or a potential source of further information does not mean that the author or the publisher endorses the information the organization or Website may provide or recommendations it may make. Further, readers should be aware that Internet Websites listed in this work may have changed or disappeared between when this work was written and when it is read. No warranty may be created or extended by any promotional statements for this work. Neither the publisher nor the author shall be liable for any damages arising herefrom.

Library of Congress Cataloging-in-Publication Data
De Brún, Caroline.
  Searching skills toolkit : finding the evidence / by Caroline De Brún, Nicola Pearce-Smith ; edited by Carl
Heneghan, Rafael Perera, Douglas Badenoch.
    p. ; cm.
  ISBN 978-1-4051-7888-4
  1. Systematic reviews (Medical research)--Handbooks, manuals, etc. 2. Database searching--Handbooks,
manuals, etc. 3. Evidence-based medicine--Handbooks, manuals, etc. I. Pearce-Smith, Nicola. II. Heneghan,
Carl. III. Perera, Rafael. IV. Badenoch, Douglas. V. Title.
  [DNLM: 1. Information Storage and Retrieval--methods--Handbooks. 2. Databases as Topic--Handbooks. 3.
Evidence-Based Medicine--Handbooks. 4. Internet--Handbooks. W 49 D278s 2009]
  R853.S94D4 2009
  616.0072--dc22

                                                                                          2008030327

ISBN: 978-1-4051-7888-4

A catalogue record for this book is available from the British Library.

Set in 7.75/9.75 pt Helvetica by Sparks, Oxford – www.sparkspublishing.com

Printed and bound in Singapore by Ho Printing Singapore pte Ltd

1 2009

Table of Contents

1. Introduction

The concept 'evidence-based medicine' was first used by David Sackett and colleagues at McMaster University in Ontario, Canada, in the early 1990s. It means

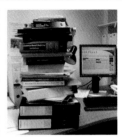

'…the integration of best research evidence with clinical expertise and patient values.'[1]

Thus the aim of evidence-based practice (EBP) is to improve the quality of information on which decisions are made.

EBP provides resources to help health professionals find the best-quality information to answer their clinical questions. Without these resources, health professionals become overloaded with information, and don't have the time to appraise all the current material published.

In 1972, Archie Cochrane, a British epidemiologist, became concerned that most decisions about interventions were based on an unstructured selection of information, of varying quality.

When making choices at home, such as what car to buy, we usually do some background research, for example ask friends, look at car magazines, watch television programmes about cars, etc. We don't have all the answers, not as professionals and not as human beings. We may have gut instincts to guide us, and these can be useful. But you cannot base your choice on gut instinct. Intuition based on professional expertise is part of the evidence-based practice concept, and can be applied to patient care, as long as it is supported by the best available research evidence.

Why search?

Searching skills are a necessity for all clinicians who want to stay up to date with best practice. Given the vast increase in research publication and the improved access to research via open access journals, health professionals

---

1   Sackett DL, Strauss SE, Richardson WS, Rosengerg W, Haynes RB. *Evidence-based Medicine: How to Practice and Teach EBM*. Edinburgh: Churchill Livingstone, 2000.

need to know where and how to find the best evidence. In 1999 there were an estimated 32 000 medical journals around the world;[2] the medical literature expands at a rate of 7% per year, doubling approximately every 10–15 years.[3] Currently 400 000 articles are added to the biomedical literature each year.[4]

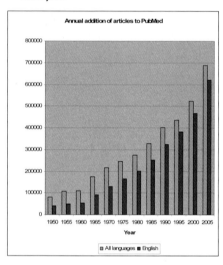

Of note, 50 years ago the majority of research was published in languages other than English, whereas currently almost 90% of articles are published in English.

Open access resources, such as Biomed Central (www.biomedcentral.com), provide access to 190 peer-reviewed journals covering a range of health-related specialties.

Reading and reviewing all the literature is not feasible for anyone, let alone busy health professionals. There is a range of resources available to help health professionals find the relevant information they require, but some sources contain better-quality information and should be targeted first.

2   Library and Information Statistics Unit. *Library and Information Statistics Tables, 1998*. Loughborough, UK: University of Loughborough, 1999.

3   Price DS. The development and structure of the biomedical literature. In: Warren KS (ed.) *Coping with the Biomedical Literature: A Primer for the Scientist and Clinicians*. Praeger, 1981.

4   Davis DA, Ciurea I, Flanagan TM, Perrier L. Solving the information overload problem: a letter from Canada. Med J Australia 2004;180(6 Suppl.),S68–S71.

Evidence-based practice requires time and a resource investment as there is so much research to read to inform practice. The aim of this Search Skills Toolkit is to show you the tools for finding the best available evidence faster and more efficiently.

The toolkit has been divided up into chapters covering the basic skills and information you need to know to be an effective searcher. You may wish to work through the chapters in order, but for a quick overview we recommend starting with Chapter 2. This chapter outlines where to go to conduct a health information search, depending on how much time you have, what type of publication you require or the specific topic area. Where appropriate, references are given directing you to the essential chapters you need to read.

When you see this symbol

Chapter 8 Refining research

it is directing you to more information in another chapter.

This note is alerting you to sites we have found particularly useful and would definitely recommend.

Recommend this site to a friend

Keeping up to date

You probably meet your current information needs by a variety of strategies:
- Toss a coin (may be useful if there are only two options and you already know both).
- Guess, fine if you have the confidence, but what if you're asked to justify your decision?
- 'Do no harm', i.e. don't try anything dangerously innovative!
- Remember what you learned during your professional training, which was considered optimum treatment 10 years ago.
- Ask colleagues (but if you ask three people, you may well get three opinions, so who is correct?).
- Textbooks: how old are your textbooks and how decayed was the material in them when you bought them?
- Browse journals: getting better, but which ones do you choose?
- Searching bibliographic databases.

Apparently doctors use some two million pieces of information to manage patients. Textbooks, journals and other existing information tools are not adequate for answering the questions that arise: textbooks are out of date, and 'the signal to noise' ratio of journals is too low for them to be useful in daily practice. When you see a patient you usually generate at least one question; more questions arise than a doctor seems to recognize. Most questions concern treatment, some are highly complex. Many questions go unanswered, the main reason being lack of time. Doctors very rarely consider using formal electronic searches.

Consider how you currently keep up to date
- *Write down one recent patient problem.*
- *What was the critical question?*
- *Did you answer it? If so, how?*

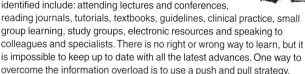

Reflect on how you learn and keep up to date. How much time do you spend on each process? Activities usually identified include: attending lectures and conferences, reading journals, tutorials, textbooks, guidelines, clinical practice, small group learning, study groups, electronic resources and speaking to colleagues and specialists. There is no right or wrong way to learn, but it is impossible to keep up to date with all the latest advances. One way to overcome the information overload is to use a push and pull strategy.

The 'push' method is the information we gather from the variety of sources that we receive across a wide spectrum of topics. This could be lectures, seminars, reading journals and magazines, or listening to Richard and Judy. To improve on this technique you should consider reading some pre-appraised source material. An example is the EBM journal or Clinical Evidence, this will cut down the time you spend allowing for more leisure activities.

The second method is the 'pull' technique, whereby you keep a record of the questions you formulate using the PICO principle (see page 38), and then 'pull' information as you need it. Clinical Evidence can be used for this sort of information gathering, but the use of a formal literature search would be more useful in obtaining an answer.

2. Where to start?

The essentials of searching the literature

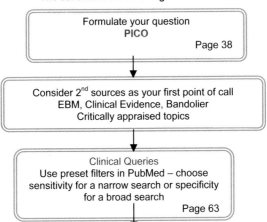

Formulate your question
PICO
Page 38

Consider 2nd sources as your first point of call
EBM, Clinical Evidence, Bandolier
Critically appraised topics

Clinical Queries
Use preset filters in PubMed – choose
sensitivity for a narrow search or specificity
for a broad search
Page 63

For articles on therapy consider the Cochrane Database of Systematic
Reviews as your first point of call. However, you can access these by getting
to grips with PubMed clinical queries and using the systematic review filter.

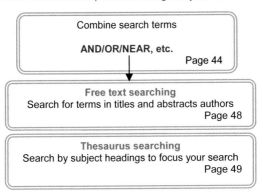

Combine search terms

AND/OR/NEAR, etc.
Page 44

Free text searching
Search for terms in titles and abstracts authors
Page 48

Thesaurus searching
Search by subject headings to focus your search
Page 49

Limiting: Reduce the number of references by language, publication year,
publication type, etc.

Where to start?
Ask yourself:

1. How much time do I have, e.g. 5 minutes or 1 hour?
2. What type of publication am I looking for, e.g. a guideline or a systematic review?
3. Is my query about a specific topic, e.g. drug or safety information?

1. How much time do I have?

Quick search <5 min	See key chapter	See related chapters
1. PubMed Clinical Queries www.pubmed.gov Click on Clinical Queries *Recommend this site to a friend*	**Chapter 8:** Refining search results *What is covered?* **a.** Search by clinical study type **b.** Systematic reviews **c.** Specific and sensitive searches	**Chapter 5:** Formulating clinical questions **Chapter 9:** Searching specific healthcare databases **Appendix 1:** Ten tips for effective searching
2. Secondary sources **a.** Clinical guidelines www.nice.org.uk **b.** EBM summaries www.ebm.bmj.com **c.** Subject gateways www.tripdatabase.com **d.** Systematic reviews www.cochrane.org	**Chapter 3:** Sources of clinical information: an overview *What is covered?* Web addresses, search examples for EB secondary sources	**Chapter 5:** Formulating clinical questions
3. The Internet (World Wide Web) Search engines, e.g. Google www.google. co.uk	**Chapter 4:** Using search engines on the World Wide Web *What is covered?* **a.** Advantages and disadvantages **b.** Search engines **c.** Using keywords, phrases **d.** Evaluating quality	**Chapter 12:** Critical appraisal

Intermediate search <1 hour	See key chapter	See related chapters
1. Secondary sources **a.** Clinical guidelines www.nice.org.uk **b.** EBM summaries www.ebm.bmj.com **c.** Subject gateways www.tripdatabase.com **d.** Systematic reviews www.cochrane.org	**Chapter 3:** Sources of clinical information: an overview *What is covered?* Details, web addresses, search examples for EB secondary sources	**Chapter 5:** Formulating clinical questions
2. PubMed www.pubmed.gov	**Chapter 9:** Searching specific healthcare databases *What is covered?* **a.** Search effectively using free text and MeSH **b.** Combine search terms with Boolean **c.** Limit your search **d.** View and save results **e.** Use features of PubMed	**Chapter 5:** Formulating clinical questions **Chapter 6:** Building a search strategy **Chapter 7:** Free text versus thesaurus **Chapter 8:** Refining search results **Appendix 1:** Ten tips for effective searching
3. Systematic search using other healthcare databases **a.** CINAHL **b.** EMBASE	**Chapter 9:** Searching specific healthcare databases *What is covered?* How to: **a.** Search effectively using free text and thesaurus **b.** Combine search terms with Boolean **c.** View and save results	**Chapter 6:** Building a search strategy **Chapter 7:** Free text versus thesaurus **Chapter 11:** Saving/ recording citations for future use **Appendix 1:** Ten tips for effective searching

Comprehensive search	See key chapters	See related chapters
1. Secondary sources **a.** Clinical guidelines **b.** Systematic reviews (from Cochrane, PubMed)	**Chapter 3:** Sources of clinical information: an overview **Chapter 9:** Searching specific healthcare databases *What is covered?* **a.** Details and web addresses for EB secondary sources **b.** PubMed and the Cochrane Library	**Chapter 5:** Formulating clinical questions
2. Systematic search using healthcare databases **a.** MEDLINE **b.** CINAHL **c.** EMBASE	**Chapter 9:** Searching specific healthcare databases *What is covered?* **a.** Effectively using free text and thesaurus **b.** Combine search terms with Boolean **c.** View and save results	**Chapter 3:** Sources of clinical information: an overview **Chapter 7:** Free text versus thesaurus **Chapter 11:** Saving/recording citations for future use **Appendix 1:** Ten tips for effective searching
3. Citation pearl searching	**Chapter 10:** Citation pearl searching *What is covered?* **a.** Related links in PubMed **b.** Similar pages in Google **c.** Author search **d.** Keyword search	

2. What type of publication am I looking for?

Many focused clinical questions allow you to see what type of research study you need to answer your question. Many databases provide a 'Clinical Query' service, which uses in-built filters to limit your search so that you only find systematic reviews or randomized controlled trials. PubMed Clinical Queries is a good example of this service.

Chapter 8 Refining research results

Sources on the Internet for finding different publication types

Before you start it is important to recognize – just like the wise owl – what type of publication is most appropriate to answer your question; for example, for a therapeutic intervention you may look at a systematic review.

Guidelines: these are formal documents that have been developed by a group of professionals, so that other health professionals know what the best practice is for a procedure. The AGREE Instrument is a tool for appraising guidelines: www.agreecollaboration.org/instrument/.

National Library of Guidelines
www.library.nhs.uk/guidelinesfinder/

National Guideline Clearinghouse
(This also has a feature that lets you compare searches)
www.guideline.gov/

Professional organizations
(such as Royal Colleges and National Associations, etc.)
www.ipl.org/div/subject/browse/hea00.00.00/

Systematic reviews: these collect and critically appraise all studies on a particular topic, providing a thorough and structured summary of what is known and what is not known. A meta-analysis is a summary of the results. The following are the recommended sources for finding systematic reviews:

Cochrane Library
www.thecochranelibrary.org

PubMed Clinical Queries
www.ncbi.nlm.nih.gov/entrez/query/static/clinical.shtml#reviews

National Library for Health Specialist Libraries
www.library.nhs.uk/specialistlibraries/

Patient information: Patients need to know where to find the best information available to them. When using health information from Internet sources that have not been validated, use Discern (www.discern.org.uk), an online checklist for people to use to help them evaluate the quality of a site. The tool contains a list of questions to ask when looking at a site.

Health On the Net Foundation
www.hon.ch/

NHS Choices
www.nhs.uk/Conditions/Pages/bodymap.aspx

Consumer and Patient Health Information Section (CAPHIS)
http://caphis.mlanet.org/consumer/

New York Online Access to Health (NOAH)
www.noah-health.org/en/search/health.html

Randomized controlled trials:

Cochrane Library
www.thecochranelibrary.org

PubMed Clinical Queries
www.ncbi.nlm.nih.gov/entrez/query/static/clinical.shtml

Clinical databases
AMED, CINAHL, EMBASE, MEDLINE, PsycINFO

Trial registers
Current Controlled Trials - www.controlled-trials.com/
ClinicalTrials.gov – http://clinicaltrials.gov
MRC Clinical Trials Unit - www.ctu.mrc.ac.uk/
National Cancer Institute - www.cancer.gov/clinicaltrials/search

If you are not sure about the publication type, the following is a list of all the recommended resources that may help in finding the evidence:

Subject gateways
Intute: www.intute.ac.uk/healthandlifesciences/medicine
National Library for Health: www.library.nhs.uk
National Library of Medicine: www.nlm.nih.gov/
Pinakes: www.hw.ac.uk/libwww/irn/pinakes/pinakes.html
SUMSearch: http://sumsearch.uthscsa.edu/
TRIP Database: www.tripdatabase.com/

Search engines (use with caution and appraise results)
AltaVista: www.av.com
Google: www.google.com
Google Scholar: http://scholar.google.co.uk/
Yahoo: www.yahoo.co.uk

3. Is my query about a specific topic?

When searching the World Wide Web, it is important to maintain a list of high-quality resources. There are tools for storing and sharing favourite web resources and these are described in Chapter 4, *Using search engines on the World Wide Web.*

Topic	Resource
Drug information	UK: www.bnf.org US: www.fda.gov/ Merck manual: www.merck.com/mmpe/index.html
Safety information	UK: www.mhra.gov.uk/index.htm US: www.fda.gov/cder/index.html Europe: www.emea.europa.eu/home.htm WHO: www.who.int/medicines/en/
Subject specific e.g. cancer, diabetes, mental health	UK specialist libraries* www.library.nhs.uk/specialistlibraries/
Health services	UK: www.nhs.uk US: www.hhs.gov/ WHO: www.who.int/en/
Health statistics	UK: www.statistics.gov.uk/ US: www.cdc.gov/nchs/ Australia: www.aihw.gov.au/ WHO: www.who.int/whosis/en/ by country: www.who.int/countries/en/ e.g. China: www.who.int/countries/chn/en/

*There are numerous subject-specific sites to search. You will find information through charities (e.g. British Heart Foundation: www.bhf.org.uk/), patient groups (e.g. Anticoagulation Europe: www.anticoagulationeurope.org/) or through clinician associations (e.g. American Health Association: www.americanheart.org/).

3. Sources of clinical information: an overview

There is a wide range of clinical information sources available to health professionals and patients – these sources may be in the form of books, journals, conference proceedings, Internet sites, etc. Some sources will be reliable but others may contain poor-quality information. Finding the best evidence requires knowledge of the most appropriate sources. This section describes the most useful sources of good-quality health information.

Medical libraries

You may want to consider involving a search specialist in some of your searches. For some studies (e.g. systematic reviews) you should consider them as an essential part of the project.

We use search specialists for the following:

- Specialist collections – databases, books and journals.
- Accessing full-text articles – sometimes the easiest way to get an article is to email your librarian.
- Development and undertaking of detailed search protocols in systematic reviews – it is worth considering involving a search specialist from the outset when undertaking a systematic review.
- For teaching and running workshops on search skills.

The Internet

Many people use the Internet to find information, particularly when they need it quickly. There are good points and bad points associated with finding information this way. Known as the World Wide Web ('www'), the Internet is a vast collection of reliable and unreliable information, personal opinion, expertise, facts, etc.

Internet searching where do you start?

Try to make sure you are using good-quality resources, or that you use procedures for evaluating the quality of the results. Listed below are Internet sources that can be used to find clinical information, in order of reliability.

Sources containing secondary evidence

Secondary evidence draws together a range of primary research in the form of an overview or structured summary. Forms of secondary evidence include:

- systematic reviews
- critical reviews
- structured abstracts, with or without expert commentaries

Systematic reviews are available via the Cochrane Library (www.cochrane. org/index.htm). The abstracts of Cochrane reviews can also be browsed and searched from the Cochrane Collaboration site.

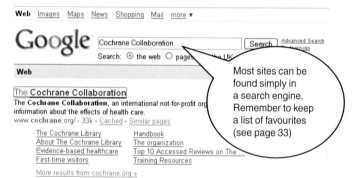

Most sites can be found simply in a search engine. Remember to keep a list of favourites (see page 33)

Worked example: Find a Cochrane systematic review on the treatment of hypertension associated with heart disease.

1. Go to the Browse abstracts page of the Cochrane Collaboration (www.cochrane.org/reviews/index.htm).
2. Type in search terms, e.g. heart disease hypertension.
3. Click Search Reviews.
4. Abstracts of Cochrane systematic reviews are displayed.
5. If you have access to the full text from the Cochrane Library, you can click through directly to the desired review.

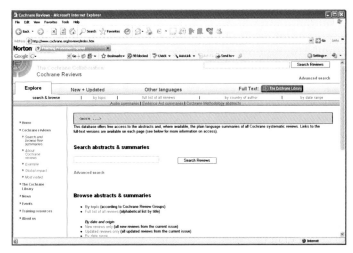

The Database of Abstracts of Reviews of Effectiveness (DARE) also contains good-quality systematic reviews, most of which contain structured abstracts and commentaries from the York Centre for Reviews and Dissemination (CRD) team: www.crd.york.ac.uk/crdweb/

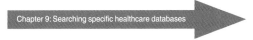

Chapter 9: Searching specific healthcare databases

Journals containing informative abstracts with expert commentaries include:
- *Evidence-Based Medicine* http://ebm.bmj.com/
- *Evidence-Based Nursing* http://ebn.bmj.com/
- *Evidence-Based Mental Health* http://ebmh.bmj.com/
- *Evidence-Based Dentistry* www.nature.com/ebd/index.html
- *Evidence-Based Complementary and Alternative Medicine* http://ecam. oxfordjournals.org/
- *International Journal of Evidence-Based Healthcare* www. blackwellpublishing.com/journal.asp?ref=1744-1595
- *POEMs (Patient-Oriented Evidence that Matters)* www.pjonline.com/ noticeboard/series/poem.html
- *Bandolier* www.jr2.ox.ac.uk/Bandolier/
- *BMJ Clinical Evidence* www.clinicalevidence.com/
- *ACP Journal Club* www.acpjc.org/

Guidelines databases

For UK guidance, use the National Library of Guidelines (www.library.nhs.uk/
guidance/). It is based on the guidelines produced by the National Institute for
Health and Clinical Excellence (NICE) and other national agencies.

- National Library of Guidelines
  www.library.nhs.uk/guidelinesFinder/

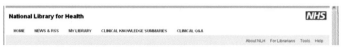

International guidelines are available from:
- US National Guideline Clearinghouse
  www.guideline.gov/

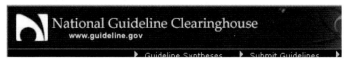

- US Agency for Healthcare Research and Quality
  www.ahrq.gov/
- New Zealand Guidelines Group – Guidelines Library
  www.nzgg.org.nz/
- Australian National Health and Medical Research Council
  www.nhmrc.gov.au/
- WHO programes and projects
  www.who.int/entity/en/
- Appraisal of guidelines – AGREE Instrument
  www.agreecollaboration.org/instrument/
- British Columbia Ministry of Health Guidelines
  www.health.gov.bc.ca/gpac/alphabetical.html
- Institute for Clinical Systems Improvement
  www.icsi.org/guidelines_and_more/index.aspx?catID=12
- Michigan Quality Improvement Consortium Guidelines
  www.mqic.org/guid.htm

- National Institute for Health and Clinical Excellence (NICE)
  www.nice.org.uk
- Scottish Intercollegiate Guidelines Network (SIGN)
  www.sign.ac.uk/

Professional organizations

Professional organizations, such as the Royal College of Nursing, Royal College of Surgeons, Chartered Society of Physiotherapy, etc. often are working on creating guidelines that have not yet been publicized on guidelines databases.

- A list of professional organizations in the UK is provided by the University of Central England
  http://library.uce.ac.uk/hprostatu.htm
- Yahoo has created a directory of professional organizations around the world
  http://dir.yahoo.com/Health/Medicine/Organizations/Professional/
- A list of medical academies and healthcare professional associations in the USA and Canada is provided by Pam Pohly Associates
  www.pohly.com/assoc2.html

Subject gateways

These are filtered versions of search engines. They allow you to search information and websites that have met specified criteria – this avoids irrelevant sites or sites containing unreliable material. Examples of subject gateways include:

Recommend this site to a friend

- TRIP (Turning Research Into Practice) database
  www.tripdatabase.com

Worked example: Find information on the treatment of hypertension associated with heart disease

In TRIP search box, type in the search terms, e.g. 'heart disease' and hypertension and treatment. Click www.tripdatabase.com

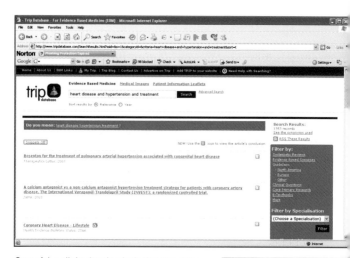

One of the slight drawbacks is that you get a lot of records for your search (2440 records in this case) if you don't know how to Boolean search. The neat thing though is that you get your results filtered by the type of evidence. For instance, you can obtain results for North American or European Guidelines.

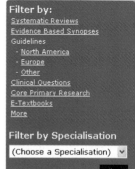

Filter by:
Systematic Reviews
Evidence Based Synopses
Guidelines
 - North America
 - Europe
 - Other
Clinical Questions
Core Primary Research
E-Textbooks
More

Filter by Specialisation
(Choose a Specialisation) ▾

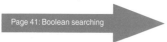

Page 41: Boolean searching

Others subject gateways to try:

- SUMSearch
  http://sumsearch.uthscsa.edu/
- Intute: health & life sciences (formerly known as BIOME) www.intute.ac.uk/healthandlifesciences/
- Pinakes Subject Launchpad (this is not clinical information, but could still be useful for background information)
  www.hw.ac.uk/libWWW/irn/pinakes/pinakes.html
- Librarians' Internet Index (a list of reliable websites)
  http://lii.org/

Online clinical databases

If nothing relevant or up to date is found from the above sources, then the next step is to search an online clinical database. These databases contain references to journal articles that have been indexed for easier retrieval. It is important to remember that the content on most databases will not have been appraised.

Recommend this site to a friend

Because the Medline database is freely available as 'PubMed' (www.pubmed.gov) from the National Library of Medicine we find it useful in daily searching. The majority of the content is only available in abstract format, but as open access publishing develops, a growing number of records are linking to freely available, full-text research papers, via PubMed Central (www.pubmedcentral.nih.gov/).

> Chapter 9: Searching specific healthcare databases

Examples of clinical databases are:

- **AMED (1985 to date)**
  This is produced by the British Library, and is available via Dialog and Ovid. It contains abstracts of articles on complementary medicines and alternative therapies.
- **CINAHL (1982 to date)**
  The Cumulative Index of Nursing and Allied Health Literature is available from EBSCO, and contains abstracts of articles on nursing and allied health disciplines, including occupational therapy, physiotherapy and dietetics.
- **EMBASE (1974 to date)**
  This is produced by Elsevier, and is available via Dialog and Ovid. It is the European version of Medline, containing abstracts of articles on medicine and pharmacology, mainly from European journals.
- **MEDLINE and PubMed (1950 to date)**
  The US National Library of Medicine produces this resource, and it is available via Dialog and Ovid.

- **PsycInfo (1887 to date)**

  The American Psychological Association produces this database, which is available via Dialog and Ovid. It contains abstracts of articles and book chapters on psychology and psychological aspects of related disciplines, such as management and learning. The coverage of this database goes back to 1887.

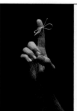

The majority of databases will cover from 5 up to 50 years back, with the exception of PsycInfo, which goes back to 1887.

There is some overlap because the databases cover similar topics, although from different points of view, i.e. nursing, psychiatry, medicine and alternative medicine. For this reason, it is essential that when carrying out a comprehensive search you MUST search MORE THAN ONE database.

When all else fails, you may need to use:

Search engines and directories

These are tools that allow you to search through the 11.5 billion web pages to find websites matching your criteria. In actual fact, no one engine searches the entire Internet.

Search engines are managed by robots, whereas directories are managed by human editors.

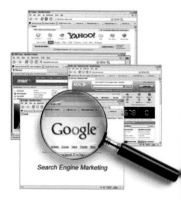

Search Engine Marketing

Google (www.google.co.uk), AltaVista (http://uk.altavista.com/) and MSN (http://uk.msn.com/) are examples of search engines, whereas Yahoo (www.yahoo.co.uk) is a good example of a directory. The benefit of using a directory is that the content has been organized, so it is easier to browse and find.

Problems with web information and search engines:
- Users rarely go past the first page of hits on search engines such as Google
- Advertisers buy prominence on websites, in news media and in search engines
- There are no controls over quality
- Information is highly likely to be biased
- Authorship and currency may be hard to determine
- Reliability is not the same as popularity nor, indeed, notoriety

---

Using a search engine requires the input of appropriate keywords and spellings. They all follow the same principles of searching – that is, type in a keyword or phrase. But because they are all competitors, they have all been developed by different organizations, and so they will have developed their own special search features and shortcuts. Because of this, although they all have the same goal – to find information – there will always be differences in the way they operate. So, when searching the Internet, it is worth looking at the 'Help' page, which each search engine will have, to identify best practice for searching that resource.

Many search engines will also have an 'Advanced Search' feature that enables you to limit and refine your search by year, by country, by language, etc. Limiting is vital when searching the Internet, because so many results will be retrieved.

The results that are retrieved will vary in content, authorship, currency and, most importantly, quality. Anyone can put content on the Internet, but not everyone is an expert. It is vital to be aware of this, particularly when searching for high-quality evidence.

If searching the Internet via search engines is the only option, there are some useful websites that can help identify quality sites or facilitate the quality evaluation process of a website.

There are many more search engines available. 'Search Engine Watch' describes the differences between the different search engines (http://searchenginewatch.com/showPage.html?page=2156221).

Chapter 4: Using search engines on the World Wide Web

Networks and/or colleagues

There are many clinical networks where people working with a similar goal can share ideas and learn from each other; likewise, the local networks in which you practice. You must be aware of the potential biases when asking colleagues, as they might not be expert in the field or the knowledge they have may be too localized or out of date. Formal networks are available:

The Cochrane Collaboration has groups and centres around the world. Each group has a web page so that you can see what work is in progress (cochrane.org/contact/index.htm).

CHAINs (Contact, Help, Advice and Information Networks) are online networks for people working in health and social care. They are based around specific areas of interest, and give people a simple and informal way of contacting each other to exchange ideas and share knowledge.

JBI-CHAIN International
www.joannabriggs.edu.au/about/chain_international.php
JBI-CHAIN Australia
www.joannabriggs.edu.au/about/chain_australia.php
CHAIN Canada
www.epoc.uottawa.ca/CHAINCanada/
CHAIN England
http://chain.ulcc.ac.uk/chain/

Other key Internet sources of information

There is so much information on the Internet, it is essential to have a list of trusted websites to hand (the easiest way is to keep a list of 'Favourites' on Internet Explorer, or a similar browser). The following is a list of additional Internet sites for a range of disciplines and languages:

Allied health
*   Intute – Internet for Nursing
    www.vts.intute.ac.uk/he/tutorial/nurse/
*   PEDro – Physiotherapy Evidence Database
    www.pedro.fhs.usyd.edu.au/
*   PEDro – Physiotherapy Evidence Database - German version
    www.pedro.fhs.usyd.edu.au/german/index_german.html

Cross-discipline

- askMedline
  http://askmedline.nlm.nih.gov/ask/ask.php
- Bandolier
  www.jr2.ox.ac.uk/bandolier/

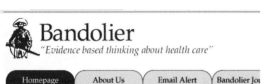

- Best BETs
  www.bestbets.org/
- British Medical Journal ABC series
  http://resources.bmj.com/bmj/topics/abcs
- BMJ Clinical Evidence useful links
  http://clinicalevidence.bmj.com/ceweb/resources/useful_links.jsp
- Campbell Collaboration
  www.campbellcollaboration.org/
- ClinicalTrials.gov
  http://clinicaltrials.gov/
- Current Controlled Trials
  www.controlled-trials.com/
- Intute – Health and Life Sciences (formerly OMNI – Organised Medical Networked Information)
  www.intute.ac.uk/healthandlifesciences/medicine/
- Medhunt – from Health On the Net Foundation (HON)
  www.hon.ch/MedHunt/
- SUMSearch
  http://sumsearch.uthscsa.edu/

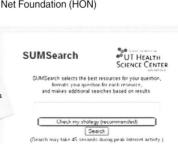

Midwifery and nursing

- Intute – Midwifery
  www.vts.intute.ac.uk/he/tutorial/nurse/
- Joanna Briggs Institute for Evidence-Based Nursing and Midwifery
  www.joannabriggs.edu.au/about/home.php
- Evidence-Based Practice
  http://evidence.ahc.umn.edu/ebn.htm
- Evidence-Based Nursing
  http://hsl.mcmaster.ca
- Evidence-Based Nursing Tools
  http://muhc-ebn.mcgill.ca/EBN_tools.htm
- Introduction to Evidence-Based Nursing
  www.cebm.utoronto.ca/syllabi/nur/intro.htm
- NAP (Nursing, Midwifery and Allied Health gateway)
  www.intute.ac.uk/healthandlifesciences/nursing/
- Journal of Evidence-Based Nursing
  http://ebn.bmj.com/

Public health

- CDC (Centers for Disease Control and Prevention) WONDER
  (Wide-ranging Online Data for Epidemiologic Research) database
  http://wonder.cdc.gov

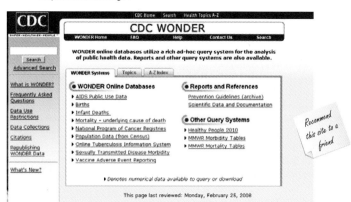

- Centers for Disease Control and Prevention
  www.cdc.gov
- E-Roadmap to Evidence-Based Public Health Practice
  www.publichealthsolutions.org/

- Evidence-Based Practice for Public Health
  http://library.umassmed.edu/ebpph/index.cfm
- Evidence-Based Public Health Portal
  http://ebling.library.wisc.edu/portals/pophealth/ebph.cfm
- National Library for Public Health
  www.library.nhs.uk/publichealth/
- Popline – connecting the world's reproductive health literature
  http://db.jhuccp.org/ics-wpd/popweb/basic.html
- Public Health's Digital Library for Seattle and King County
  www.metrokc.gov/health/library/evidence.htm
- WHO Global Health Atlas
  http://who.int/GlobalAtlas
- World Health Organization
  www.who.int

Patient information
- CAPHIS (Consumer and Patient Health Information Section)
  http://caphis.mlanet.org/consumer/
- EQUIP – foreign language patient information
  www.equip.nhs.uk/language.html
- Health On the Net Foundation
  www.hon.ch/
- Henry Ford Health System Health Encyclopedia
  www.henryford.com/body.cfm?id=39115
- Henry Ford Health System Patient Information
  www.henryford.com/myhealth/adamdisplay_bguide.cfm
- New York Online Access to Health
  www.noah-health.org/en/search/health.html
- NHS Choices
  www.nhs.uk/Conditions/Pages/bodymap.aspx

Miscellaneous
- EBM glossary
  www.cebm.net/
- EBM terms
  www.cebm.utoronto.ca/glossary/index.htm#top

Formulating clinical questions
- PubMed PICO
  http://pubmedhh.nlm.nih.gov/nlm/pico/piconew.html
- The well-built clinical question
  http://umanitoba.ca/faculties/medicine/units/family_medicine/media/
  APPENDICESCATassignmentAHAK.pdf

- The well-built clinical question
  www.biomed.lib.umn.edu/inst/clinicalquestion.pdf
- Where's the evidence?
  www.wherestheevidence.nhmrc.gov.au/asp/index.
  asp?sid=2228&page=questions

Non-English-language sites

Healthcare is international, and there are many quality health resources
available in different languages:

Chinese:

- Cochrane Collaboration
  www.cochrane.org/index_zh.htm

French:

- Catalogue et Index des Sites Médicaux Francophones (CISMeF)
  www.cismef.org/
- Cochrane Collaboration
  www.cochrane.org/index_fr.htm
- Critique et pratique
  http://machaon.fmed.ulaval.ca/medecine/cetp/

German:

- Cochrane Collaboration
  www.cochrane.org/index_de.htm
- Deutsches Netzwerk Evidenzbasierte Medizin e.V.
  www.ebm-netzwerk.de/
- Horten-Zentrum für praxisorientierte Forschung und Wissenstransfer
  www.evimed.ch/

Italian:

- Gruppo Italiano per la Medicina Basata sulle Evidenze
  http://www.gimbe.org/

Japan:

- Evidence-Based Medicine – Japan
  www.med.nihon-u.ac.jp/department/public_health/ebm/

Russian:

- Cochrane Collaboration
  www.cochrane.org/index_ru.htm

Spanish:

- Atrapando la evidencia
  www.infodoctor.org/rafabravo/netting.htm
- Bandolera - Bandolier in Spanish
  www.infodoctor.org/bandolera/

- Clinical question formulation – Spanish
  www.fisterra.com/mbe/mbe_temas/12/preguntas.htm
- Cochrane Collaboration
  www.cochrane.org/index_es.htm
- Instituto Argentino de Medicina Basada en las Evidencias
  www.iambe.org.ar/
- CASPe
  www.redcaspe.org/homecasp.asp

Programa de habilidades
en lectura crítica
España

Inicio | Contactos | Enlaces | Herramientos | Próximos Talleres | Mapa de la web | Buscador

Recommend
this site to a
friend

4. Using search engines on the World Wide Web

The Web is a vast collection of knowledge and information on all topics, created by a range of authors, both expert and non-expert. With this in mind, it is difficult to gauge the quality of the content found on the Internet, particularly when searching for health-related information. This section will highlight the good and bad points of searching the World Wide Web.

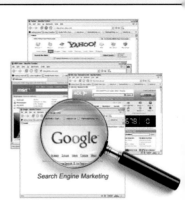

Search Engine Marketing

Advantages	Disadvantages
The World Wide Web is available 24 hours a day, 7 days a week	There is no guarantee of quality, accuracy or reliability because anybody can write for the World Wide Web, be they expert or amateur
Information can be very up to date	Unless the site is maintained on a regular basis, the information can quickly go out of date
Access is available to full-text and unpublished information	Different search methods can make it difficult to find the information required

Search engines
Search engines allow you to search billions of pages on the World Wide Web. All search engines require the input of appropriate keywords or phrases. For example, if you want to find some information on clinical trials in diabetes for children, your keywords would be: diabetes, children, clinical trials. Typing these keywords into Google (www.google.co.uk)

quickly retrieves web pages containing all the above words – note that the search retrieves over *1 million* results.

You can use phrase searching to reduce the number of pages retrieved; for example, typing: diabetes children 'clinical trials', will only retrieve pages with the exact phrase 'clinical trials', as well as the words diabetes and children.

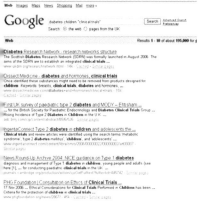

On Google this reduces the hits, but still retrieves around 200 000. Using a search engine will invariably retrieve tens of thousands of results, so try to use as many keywords as possible.

The quality of the material found on the web varies enormously, so you should consider any information carefully before using it.

Using a general search engine for finding health information is not generally recommended as a first port of call unless the subject is very rare, or you want to do some background research to get ideas for a more focused search.

Evaluating material found on the World Wide Web
Researchers should be aware of some of the pitfalls involved with searching the Internet. Silberg et al. (1997) published some guidance on appraising material found on the Internet. Simple questions should be considered, such as:

1. Authorship – Who wrote the research? Are they qualified? Where has the funding come from? Is there any bias?
2. Attribution – Is there any copyright information on the website? What is the source of the information?

3. Disclosure – Is it clear who owns the website? Could it be an organization with a conflict of interest, e.g. medical supplier?
4. Currency – Is it clear when the research was written?
5. Content – Is it relevant to the population being researched? Is it accurate?

Anyone with a computer and access to some 'web space' can create a website to put up information on any topic. This information will be of a variable quality as the Internet has no quality control mechanisms. Therefore, information found on the Internet, especially about health and medical issues, should never be taken at face value. Some assessment of the validity and reliability of the information should be undertaken.

There are various evaluated, published criteria that can be used to help you assess the quality of health information found on websites, some of which are listed below:

DISCERN instrument – Fifteen questions to assess the quality of written information on treatment choices for a health problem:
www.discern.org.uk/
Health on the Net Code of Conduct (HONcode) – Eight principles for assessing the quality and trustworthiness of health information on the Internet
www.hon.ch/HONcode/Conduct.html
Intute: Health and Life Sciences Evaluation Guidelines – Guidelines for evaluating health and life sciences websites
www.intute.ac.uk/healthandlifesciences/IntuteHLS_Evaluation_Guidelines.doc

These, or similar criteria, should be used to assess any medical or health information found from unappraised website sources, such as those sites retrieved in a general search of the Internet using Google or Yahoo.

Hints and tips for using the World Wide Web

Tutorials
Good tutorials are often available with websites that are specifically designed to search for information, such as search engines and clinical

databases. PubMed, the database of medical citations, has a tutorial available (www.nlm.nih.gov/bsd/disted/pubmedtutorial/010_020.html).

The Cochrane Library has available a range of help sheets in different languages (www3.interscience.wiley.com/cgi-bin/mrwhome/106568753/HELP_Cochrane.html).

Advanced search facility

Many search engines have an advanced search facility that allows the application of limits to the search, enabling you to narrow by type of publication (e.g. randomized controlled trial), date of publication, country, language, organization type, etc. This enables you to refine your search when presented with overwhelming results.

For Google:

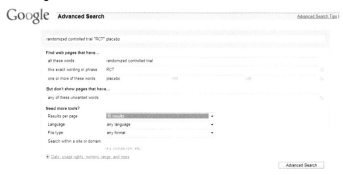

With Advanced Search you can limit your search to pages:

- that contain ALL the search terms you type in
- that contain the exact phrase you type in
- that contain at least one of the words you type in
- that do NOT contain any of the words you type in
- created in a certain file format
- that have been updated within a certain period of time
- that contain numbers within a certain range
- within a certain domain, or website

If a word is essential to getting the results you want add a '+' sign immediately in front of it in the search box. (Be sure also to include a space between the '+' sign and any other words in your search.)

For example, here's how to ensure that Google includes the 'II' in a search for *Angiotensin II* (inhibitors):

Angiotensin +II	Google Search

Synonym search

If you want to search not only for your search term but also for its synonyms, place the tilde sign ('~') immediately in front of your search term.

For example, here's how to search for cholesterol-lowering therapy information:

~cholesterol ~lipid	Google Search

Domain search

If you want to search only within one specific website, enter the search terms you're looking for, followed by the word 'site' and a colon followed by the domain name.

For example, here's how you'd find admission information on the University of Oxford site:

admission site:w w w .ox.ac.uk	Google Search

For Yahoo:

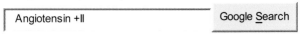

YAHOO! SEARCH _____ Yahoo! · Search Home · Help
UK–IRELAND

Advanced Web Search

You can use the options on this page to create a very specific search. Just fill in the fields you need for your current search.   [Yahoo! Search]

Show results with

	all of these words	yahoo		any part of the page ▼
	the exact phrase			any part of the page ▼
	any of these words			any part of the page ▼
	none of these words			any part of the page ▼

Tip: Use these options to look for an exact phrase or to exclude pages containing certain words. You can also limit your search to certain parts of pages.

Updated

anytime ▼

Site/Domain

◉ Any domain
○ Only .com domains   ○ Only .edu domains
○ Only .gov domains   ○ Only .org domains
○ Only .co.uk domains   ○ Only .ie domains

○ only search in this domain/site: [   ]

Tip: You can search for results in a specific website (e.g. yahoo.com) or top-level domains (e.g. .com, .org, .gov).

Yahoo has a similar facility for advance searching and also useful tick boxes to distinguish between site/domains.

Saving useful websites

When searching the World Wide Web, it is important to maintain a list of high-quality resources. There are two ways to do this:

Favourites or bookmarks

Your Internet browser, be it Internet Explorer or Firefox, will have a facility allowing you to save important web addresses, or URLs. This means that you don't have to keep on typing in the address when you want to access that page. Internet Explorer calls this facility 'Add to favourites' and it looks like this:

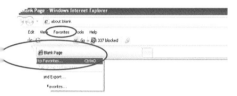

Firefox calls this facility '*Bookmarks*' and it looks like this:

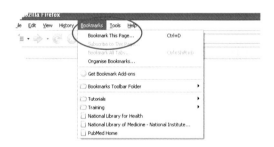

Within these facilities, you can organize your favourites into folders, naming them to suit your preferences. There is also the option to have your key resources visible on a toolbar on your browser.

One problem with this storage facility is if you use different computers in different locations. These favourites or bookmarks stay on the computer where they have been set up.

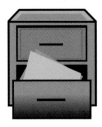

Online storage tools

To overcome this, many online tools have been developed for storing and sharing favourite web resources.

Connotea (www.connotea.org) has been developed by the Nature Publishing Group, especially for scientists and clinicians to support evidence-based medicine and knowledge sharing. This resource allows researchers to save the Internet resources they use the most, categorize them, and share them with colleagues, and then access them from whichever computer they are using. Another popular *Social Bookmarking* tool is *del.icio.us* (http://del.icio.us/).

These resources allow you to save all your favourite websites, and access them wherever you are working.

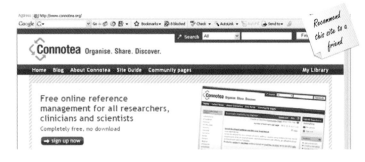

5. Formulating clinical questions

Types of question

Clinical questions may be divided into background or foreground questions. A background question asks for general knowledge about a topic, and usually involves *who, what, when, why, where* or *how*.

> **Examples of background questions:**
> *What are the side effects of taking Drug A?*
> *What causes disease B?*
> *How is virus C transmitted?*

These sorts of questions can usually be answered by using textbooks, encyclopedias, dictionaries or other reference sources.

A foreground question applies to specific patients or problems.

> **Examples of foreground questions:**
> *Will the use of acupuncture help a smoker of 30 years to quit smoking?*
> *Among children with hyperactivity disorder, does treatment with ritalin affect symptoms?*
> *What is the risk of type II diabetes for adults who are obese and take little exercise?*

Foreground questions usually need to be answered by searching primary and secondary research literature, for example journal articles and other literature indexed in medical databases and online sources.

There are four main types of foreground question that are usually asked in healthcare:

Diagnosis – how those with and without a disease or condition can be distinguished

Harm – the side effects or disadvantages to an intervention

Prognosis – how the course of the disease or condition may progress

Treatment – effectiveness of interventions such as drugs, therapies, training or provision of information

Why does this help you to search for evidence?

Knowing the type of question helps you to decide on the best type of research study to answer that question.

There are specific search terms or search filters (such as PubMed Clinical Queries) you can use for retrieving appropriate studies for each type of question.

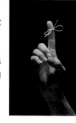

Chapter 8: Refining search results

Breaking down the clinical scenario

Searching for the answer to a clinical question – the patient story – can be complicated. By entering the entire scenario, it is unlikely that appropriate evidence will be found. The purpose of this section is to demonstrate methods for breaking down clinical scenarios to help health professionals find the best evidence available.

A clinical scenario arises from a meeting with a patient or perhaps from a gap in the research, but it is a question that is unanswered and needs to be resolved. The concept of breaking down the scenario involves identifying the keywords. This enables you to turn a complicated case description into a more manageable question, making it easier to construct an effective search strategy.

PICO[5] is a popular method of managing a clinical question. The acronym stands for:

P	Patient/Problem/Population – meaning the individual, the condition or the group that is the subject of the clinical question
I	Intervention – the treatment that might be applied to the patient, problem or population
C	Comparison – an alternative treatment that might provide similar if not greater benefits to the intervention. Please note: there may not always be a comparative intervention
O	Outcome – the expected result of the intervention

---

5   Sackett DL, Richardson WS, Rosenberg W, Haynes RB. *Evidence-based Medicine: How to Practice and Teach EBM*. New York: Churchill Livingstone, 1997.

Here is an example of a clinical scenario:

> A girl in her early twenties is being treated at your surgery for myalgic encephalomyelitis (ME). Her symptoms are extreme tiredness, pain, mood swings and night sweats. She has been prescribed Prozac, but would like to know if there are any alternative therapies that might relieve some or all of the symptoms associated with ME.

Identifying keywords

The above scenario is far too complicated to type into a search engine. No results would be retrieved. So, the first stage of the 'clinical question formulation' process is to identify the most important words – the keywords that will formulate the question. In this scenario, the keywords/phrases are underlined, as shown below:

> A **girl in her early-twenties** is being treated at your surgery for **myalgic encephalomyelitis (ME)**. Her symptoms are **extreme tiredness**, **pain**, **mood swings** and **night sweats**. She has been prescribed **Prozac**, but would like to know if there are any **alternative therapies** that might **relieve some or all of the symptoms** associated with ME.

So, from this scenario, we have:

- Age – 'girl in her early twenties' = young woman
- **P**roblem – myalgic encephalomyelitis
- **I**ntervention – Prozac
- **C**omparison – alternative medicine
- **O**utcome – relief of all or some of her symptoms

Once the keywords/phrases are identified, a **simple, focused, clinical question** can be formulated, as follows:

> A **young woman** suffering from **myalgic encephalomyelitis** has been prescribed **Prozac** but would like to know if **alternative therapies** might provide **symptom relief**.

From this clinical question, the keywords can be put into a PICO table:

Patient/Problem/	Intervention	Comparison	Outcome
Myalgic encephalomyelitis	Prozac	Alternative therapies	Symptom relief

6. Building a search strategy

Searching for evidence is a bit like going shopping. If you don't make a shopping list, you might forget to buy something you really need. When searching for evidence, if you don't make a list of all applicable terms, you might miss out on a key piece of research.

Identifying synonyms

The next stage is to compile a list of synonyms for each of the keywords. There are three things to think about:

Spelling	Research published in English may have spelling differences, depending on whether it is UK English or US English
Terminology	Different databases use different indexing terms. Medline and CINAHL indexes use the term Allied Health Personnel, whereas EMBASE uses Paramedical Personnel for the same type of health professional
Colloquial phrases	When ME was first identified, it was referred to as 'yuppie flu'. Deep vein thrombosis is sometimes referred to as 'economy class syndrome'

For a comprehensive search of the evidence, it is essential that all the alternative terms, spellings and acronyms are added to the PICO table, as shown:

P	I	C	O
Myalgic encephalomyelitis	Antidepressive agent	Alternative therapy/medicine	Symptom relief
ME	Fluoxetine	Complementary therapy/medicine	Pain relief
Post viral fatigue syndrome	Prozac	Homoeopathy	Balanced moods
Yuppie flu		Reflexology	Calm sleep
		Nutritional/diet therapy	Increase in energy levels
		Acupuncture	

Synonym sources

When looking for synonyms, you might find it useful to do some background research into the condition. Sources might include:

- Medical encyclopedias/dictionaries – looking up definitions may reveal alternative terms for the condition or symptoms.
- Colleagues – discussing the condition with colleagues, particularly those from overseas, may bring up terms that you had not thought of or perhaps not even come across before.
- Patient information – reliable patient information sources may be able to provide you with useful terms that you might want to build into your search.

Truncation and wildcards

Truncation and wildcards are handy little shortcuts, for free-text searching, which can substantially reduce the number of search terms that need to be added.

Truncation allows the use of a symbol, usually an asterisk * or a dollar sign $ to expand the search, by taking the stem of a word and adding the symbol at the end – so, child* or child$ will search for child, children, childhood, etc.

If your search involved the keyword *ulcers* or *ulceration*, you could type in *ulcer, ulcers, ulceration, ulcerated, ulcerative,* etc., or you could save time by typing in either:
- ulcer* – which searches for ulcer, ulcers, ulceration, ulcerated, ulcerative in PubMed
- ulcer$ – which searches for ulcer, ulcers, ulceration, ulcerated, ulcerative in Ovid MEDLINE and Dialog MEDLINE
- ulcer$2 – which takes the stem of the word, e.g. *ulcer,* and searches for 1- or 2-letter endings, therefore ulcer or ulcers, but not ulceration, ulcerated or ulcerative

At the end of this chapter, there is a table summarizing which forms of truncation, wildcards and Boolean operators are used by each database provider.

Truncation reduces the number of search steps, while increasing the number of hits. However, when using truncation, it is important to remember the differences in spelling. For example, the word *stabilising* could also be spelled *stabilizing,* so if you use truncation you would need to ensure that either both terms are searched for using truncation or a shorter stem is used; e.g. *stabili$* – this would look for stabilising, stabilizing and stability.

CAUTION!
Do not use too short a stem as the search will become too broad and not retrieve relevant records. For example: car* or car$ will find care, careful, cardiology, carcinogenic, etc.

Wildcards

British English and American English sometimes have different spellings, for example:

British English	**American English**
paediatric	pediatric
behaviour	behavior
colour	color

Use a **wildcard**, usually in the form of a question mark. So, instead of typing in both terms, a question mark is inserted in place of the extra letter, for example, behavio?r, colo?r, and this will search for the occurrence of the British English spelling or the American English spelling.

Wildcards are also useful for dealing with plurals, such as woman or women. You can just type wom?n to retrieve both.

NOTE!
The wildcard cannot be used near the start of a word, so when searching for oestrogen/estrogen or paediatric/pediatric, both spellings must be included.

Use the Help pages for individual databases to find out if they apply truncation and/or wildcards, and if yes, which ones they use and how.

Combining terms (also known as Boolean operators)

The process of building a search strategy involves the use of Boolean operators. These are words that combine the terms that have been selected for the search, making the search more relevant to the clinical question. Below is a summary table showing the Boolean operators available and the definition of each.

Boolean term	Definition
and/AND	Narrows the search results; all terms are searched for; e.g. measles AND children AND adults
or/OR	Broadens the search results; one or more of the search terms are found; e.g. venous thrombosis OR DVT OR deep vein thrombosis
not/NOT	Limits the searches by restricting the terminology searched for; e.g. children NOT adults
near/NEAR	Searches for all the words in a specific order, as a phrase; e.g. deep NEAR vein NEAR thrombosis. If you add a number after the word 'near', the database would search for all occurrences where the two words appear separated by the number of words matching the number; e.g. chronic NEAR3 syndrome, would find 'chronic fatigue syndrome' and 'chronic fatigue immune deficiency syndrome'
with/WITH	'With' is also referred to as 'adjacent' or 'adj'. This is useful when searching for phrases that contain smaller connecting words, such as 'of', 'the', 'by', 'for', etc. For example, community WITH1 practice will find community of practice
()	Brackets can be used in two ways: 1) When combining with two Boolean operators, e.g. measles AND (children OR adults), so the database will look for articles about children or adults with measles 2) When searching for a phrase, some databases use brackets, e.g. (assertive community treatment)
" "	By putting the keywords in inverted commas, some databases will search for the words as phrases, e.g. "assertive community treatment"

Venn diagrams of common Boolean operators:

AND

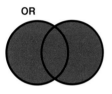

Searching for diabetes AND insulin will retrieve only those resources containing both words (the pink shaded section).

OR

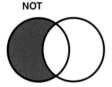

Searching for antidepressants OR counselling will retrieve resources containing either term, or both (the pink shaded section).

NOT

Searching for contraception NOT oral would exclude resources containing the word 'oral'.

WITH or ADJACENT

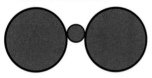

This is useful when searching for phrases using joining words, such as 'the', 'for', 'of', 'by', etc., which might usually be ignored by the database; e.g. community WITH1 practice will find research on community of practice.

NEAR

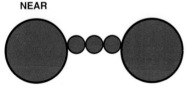

This is used to search for words in a specific order, as a phrase; e.g. deep NEAR vein NEAR thrombosis.

Some databases will insist that the Boolean operators are upper case, whereas with other databases it does not matter whether they are upper or lower case. All databases and search engines will have search tips or help pages describing the differences of their individual sites, so you can check out their policy on case sensitivity. The key point is to remember how Boolean operators are used so that you can apply them effectively.

Boolean operators are the lynch pins for the search terms, enabling you to find the most relevant references to answer your clinical questions. Some databases do use other Boolean operators, but the key ones are described here.

Table 1 specifies which databases use which Boolean operators, wildcards and truncation.

Table 1: Summary of truncation symbols, wildcards and Boolean operators (remember: each software provider has a Help facility to provide further guidance on searching)

Symbol	Definition	Cochrane	Dialog	EBSCO	OVID	PubMed	WebSPIRS
*	All words beginning with a particular stem	✓		✓		✓	✓
$	For all words beginning with a particular stem		✓		✓		
?	For all words beginning with a particular stem		✓				
?	Overcoming spelling differences and searching for singular and plurals, e.g. colo?r	✓	✓		✓		✓
:	Searches for all words beginning with a particular stem				✓		
#	Overcoming spelling differences and searching for singular and plural, e.g. colo#r				✓		
AND	For all the words	✓	✓	✓	✓	✓	✓
NOT	Excludes a word from the search	✓	✓	✓	✓	✓	✓
-	For words next to each other, in the order specified	✓	✓			✓	✓

Operator	Description					
" "	For words next to each other, in the order specified				✓	
( )	For each word and mapping to MeSH					✓
ADJ	For words next to each other, in the order specified			✓		✓
NEXT	For the 1st word with the 2nd following within the next 5 words			✓		
NEAR	For the 1st word and the 2nd in either order, within the next 5 words			✓		✓
OR	Searches for at least one of the words in the search string			✓	✓	✓
,	Can be used in place of OR			✓		
XOR	Searches for either word, but not both			✓		
WITH	Searches for all the words in the same sentence, in any order			✓		✓
SAME	Searches for all the words in the same field or paragraph, in any order			✓		
( )	For words in brackets first			✓	✓	✓
FREQ	Searches for a specified number of times the word appears in the record		✓			

··

Construction of the final search strategy

··

Using the PICO table developed at the beginning of this chapter, along with our knowledge of Boolean operators, we can now construct our search strategy in two stages.

Stage one involves combining the terms under each heading, (P, I, C and O) with 'OR'. It is not necessary to find articles containing all of these words, just articles that contain one or more of the terms.

For example:

STAGE ONE			
P	**I**	**C**	**O**
Myalgic encephalomyelitis OR ME OR Post viral fatigue syndrome OR Yuppie flu	Antidepressants OR Fluoxetine OR Prozac	Alternative therapy/ medicine OR Complementary therapy/medicine OR Homoeopathy OR Reflexology OR Nutritional/diet therapy OR Acupuncture	Symptom relief OR Pain relief OR Balanced moods OR Calm sleep OR Increase in energy levels

So, the search process would involve searching for all the terms under column P first, combining each of them with OR, and then doing the same process for columns I, C (if appropriate) and O.

Once all the terms have been combined in their groups with 'OR' you can go onto **Stage two**, which involves combining the groups (P, I, C and O) using 'AND'. If there is no comparison intervention, there will be no need to add column C into the search strategy.

STAGE TWO			
P	**I**	**C**	**O**
Myalgic encephalomyelitis	Antidepressants	Alternative therapy/ medicine	Symptom relief

AND   AND   AND

In summary, to develop an effective search strategy, you must:

1. Break down the clinical scenario and formulate a more manageable question.
2. Identify the key words and make a note of relevant synonyms.
3. Combine using appropriate Boolean concepts.

Sometimes you have to use brackets to delineate between ANDs and ORs.

P	I

(Myalgic encephalomyelitis   OR   ME   OR   Post viral fatigue syndrome

OR   Yuppie flu)

AND

(Antidepressants   OR   Fluoxetine   OR   Prozac)

Refining search strategies (also known as limiting)

In Chapter 9 there will be comprehensive descriptions for applying these search strategies to specific healthcare databases using different methods.

> Chapter 9: Searching specific healthcare databases

Once the search has been carried out, if there are too many results retrieved, the search can be further restricted with the application of limits. Limits allow the search to be restricted in a number of ways – see Chapter 8 for details.

> Chapter 8 Refining research results

7. Free text versus thesaurus

You have now completed the first three steps of the search process:

1. Formulated a searchable question
2. Identified appropriate search terms
3. Selected relevant health databases

You are now ready to search for your evidence. You can do this using:
1. Free text searching
2. Thesaurus searching

Free text

Free text, also known as 'natural language', means that the database will search for exactly what you type into the box, in any field of a record. This is the natural way to search, but not necessarily the most effective. There are pros and cons to the use of free text:

Pros	For example
Useful for unambiguous topics or new interventions not indexed elsewhere	If you type in 'assertive community treatment', the database will find papers specifically on this intervention
Brand names of drugs or proper names	If you type in Prozac, the database will find papers about Prozac
Cons	
Too many irrelevant results	If you type in diabetes, the database will search for every occurrence of the word diabetes and retrieve an unmanageable amount of results, many of which will only have a minor reference to diabetes
Disregards plurals	If you are looking for research on disability and you type in disability, the database will look for disability but not disabilities, so you will miss out on important research
Ignores spelling differences	If you are searching for papers on behaviour (British English) you will miss out on research on behavior (American English)

A more effective way of searching uses a thesaurus.

Thesaurus searching

To ensure that no literature is missed, it is important to recognize the existence of different spelling and different terminology for the same search topics. For example, deep vein thrombosis is known by many names, including DVT, economy class syndrome and venous thrombosis. Articles may use any of these words to describe DVT, and it is not always possible to second guess all the synonyms.

One way to overcome these differences when searching a database is to use the thesaurus. A thesaurus can be referred to in many ways, including:
- Medical Subject Headings (MeSH), in the database MEDLINE (see Advanced MeSH below, and Chapter 9: Searching specific healthcare databases)
- controlled vocabulary
- descriptor
- keyword
- index term

A thesaurus is a collection of terms that has been developed for a particular database – each record contained in the database is allocated several of these thesaurus terms (usually between 5 and 20) in order to identify the key themes or subjects it covers.

Example of a Medline (PubMed) record showing the MeSH terms that have been assigned to it:

MeSH Terms:
- Blood Glucose Self-Monitoring
- Diabetes Mellitus, Type 1/prevention & control
- Diabetes Mellitus, Type 2/prevention & control
- Diabetes, Gestational/prevention & control*
- Diet
- Female
- Humans
- Insulin/administration & dosage
- Patient Education as Topic*
- Pregnancy
- Prenatal Care*

This means that articles on the same topic should be allocated the same thesaurus terms, regardless of how the subject is described in the text of the article. Therefore, searching a database using specific thesaurus terms aids the retrieval of records on the same topic. The main difference with searching using thesaurus terms is that the articles you find will be specifically about the topic you are searching for – searching for a term using free text will find articles containing the word or words somewhere in the article, and will not necessarily be specifically about the topic you are interested in.

Another good reason for searching the thesaurus is that one term often incorporates a range of synonyms. For example, the MeSH term 'venous thrombosis' also searches for papers specifically on venous thromboses, deep vein thrombosis, DVT and phlebothrombosis or phlebothromboses.

Thesaurus searching also overcomes the problem of different spellings and different terminology. For example, the MeSH term Fetal Diseases, will also look for foetal diseases; moreover, the MeSH term Allied Health Personnel will retrieve Paramedical Personnel, which is the same type of health profession.

Thesaurus searching is the most efficient way of searching because you can find articles of relevance, and you save time by keying in fewer terms. However, you should be aware that the indexing of articles is subject to human error, and not all entries in a database will be correctly indexed in sufficient detail. Therefore, a combination of thesaurus and free text searching will help to prevent relevant papers being missed.

Browsing and mapping

In most databases there are two ways to use the thesaurus, browsing or automatic mapping. In PubMed you can:

1. Browse the MeSH database – this takes you to the thesaurus, and allows you to type in the term you are looking for, presenting you with a list of suitable terms. For example, typing *deep vein thrombosis* into the MeSH database will tell you that the term used in MEDLINE is '*Venous Thrombosis*'.

2. Use mapping – when you type a term into the main search box, PubMed tries automatically to map your term to an appropriate MeSH; this will then be included in your search. For example, typing *deep vein thrombosis* into the search box will automatically map to the MeSH '*Venous Thrombosis*' and include this in your search.

> **Note:** PubMed will not be able to map all terms typed into the search box to a MeSH term, so ideally you should check the MeSH database.

Advanced MeSH

MeSH terms are organized into 'trees' so that you can see how the database is applying them. An example of a MeSH tree in PubMed is shown below:

All MeSH Categories
  Diseases Category
    Cardiovascular Diseases
      Vascular Diseases
        Embolism and Thrombosis
          Thrombosis
            Venous Thrombosis
              Hepatic Vein Thrombosis
              Retinal Vein Occlusion
              Thrombophlebitis

Explode and single term
The MeSH term selected is in bold. Beneath the MeSH term, there is an indented list of narrower terms. There is an option to 'Explode' the MeSH term. This means that when the database searches for the MeSH term, it will also search for the narrower terms below the MeSH term, widening your options.

If you choose not to Explode the MeSH term, the database will only search for the single term, the MeSH term that you have typed in. This can limit too much, and it is often best to keep the search broad and narrow it down by adding more search terms.

Focus
The Focus option is not available on all databases, but it does allow you to search a particular aspect of the MeSH term that you have typed in.

Major and minor descriptors
Major descriptors are the keywords that identify the main themes of the paper. Minor descriptors are the keywords that identify the secondary themes of the paper.

Subheadings
Many databases allow you to narrow down your MeSH terms by choosing specific subheadings. Although this is a useful option, it is often best to keep the search broad and narrow it down by adding more search terms in the PICO categories.

Related terms
This is a useful feature because it allows you to see MeSH terms that might also apply to your search. For example, the related term for Fetal Diseases is Abnormalities, which you might not have thought of incorporating into your search, thinking it is too broad, but when linked to Pregnancy could bring about some appropriate results. The database does not automatically include it in the search, but you can add it.

8. Refining search results

If your search strategy has retrieved too many results, you might like to refine your search using limits or search filters. Both can be applied at the start of the search process or at the end.

Filtering search results: Limits

Once your search has been completed, many databases allow you to Limit the results using specific fields. Applying Limits reduces the amount of hits by retrieving only those records matching the chosen Limit/s.

> A field is a specific structural unit of a database record, like Title or Author.

Common fields to limit by include:

Language (.la)	Although a journal article might be in a language other than English, an English abstract is usually included, so be wary about limiting by language
Age	The major healthcare databases vary in age limits: • CINAHL: conception to approx. 6 months after delivery; conception to birth; up to 1 month old; 1–23 months; 2–5 years; 6–12 years; 13–18 years; 19–44 years; 45–64 years; 65–79 years; 80+ years • EMBASE: adults, older people, all children, children, infants, preschool children, school-age children, adolescents • Medline: all adults, adults – 19 and over; 19–44 years; 45–64 years; 65–79 years; 80 and over; all children 0–18 years; all infants birth to 23 months; birth to 1 month; 1–23 months; 2–12 years; 2–5 years; 6–12 years; 13–18 years • PsycINFO: birth to 12 years; birth to 1 month; 2–23 months; 2–5 years; 6–12 years; 13–17 years; 18 years and older; 18–29 years; 30–39 years; 40–64 years; 65 years and older; 85 years and older
Title (.ti)	Looks for your keywords only in the title of an article – this is restrictive and will miss much relevant information, but usually retrieves very relevant articles
Publication year (.py)	Retrieves all articles published in one year, or a range of years
Author (.au)	Use when searching for articles by a specific author(s)

Example 1: Ovid MEDLINE

A search limited by English language and the publication years 2005–2007:

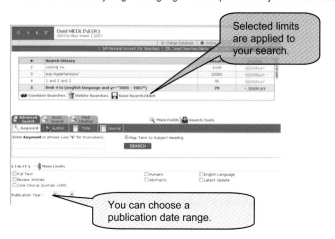

Further options to Limit can be obtained by clicking on More Limits. Other Limits include:

- Humans or Animals
- Publication Types (see further below) – as with the age groups, the major healthcare databases differ in the types of publication they offer

Worked example: PubMed

A search Limited by English language, published in the last 2 years and specific to Humans:

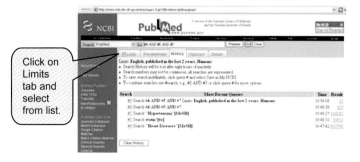

Publication Type

Limiting by attributes such as Title, Author or Date is possible as shown above, but is not the best way to limit your search if you are interested in finding better quality research studies.

One way to limit your search is to use the Publication Type field, because this allows you to search for particular study types, such as:
- Meta-Analysis
- Randomized Controlled Trial
- Clinical Trial
- Practice Guideline

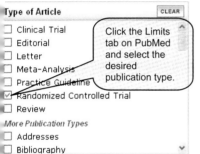

For example, if you have a Treatment/Intervention question, limit your search using the Meta-Analysis or Randomized Controlled Trial publication type on Medline.

Applying Limits within your search strategy

Limits may also be applied during your search, by typing the specific field name after your search term.

	Ovid	PubMed	Dialog
Look for the word *hypertension* in the **title**	hypertension.ti.	hypertension[ti]	hypertension.ti.
Look for records with the word *statin* in the **title** or **abstract**	statin.tw. or statin.ti,ab.	statin[tiab]	statin.ti,ab.
Look for records with *BMJ* in the **journal title**	BMJ.jn.	BMJ[ta]	BMJ.so.

....

Filtering search results: methodological filters

....

A methodological search filter is a search strategy containing search terms that relate to a research methodology (i.e. the study design). The search terms may be thesaurus (e.g. Medical Subject Headings, or MeSH), free text, publication types or a combination of all three. A filter can be used to retrieve articles of appropriate study design, to answer a particular type of question.

> You may see search filters described as:
> - 'hedges'
> - optimal search strategies
> - research methodology filters
> - Clinical Queries

A search filter may just be one or two search terms – see the table below. You can combine these single filter terms with your subject search, to assist you in finding appropriate study designs.

Question type	Best feasible study design	Best single MEDLINE search term
DIAGNOSIS	Cross-sectional study	sensitivity
HARM	Cohort study	risk
PROGNOSIS	Cohort study	Explode Cohort Studies [MeSH]
TREATMENT	Systematic review or randomized controlled trial	Meta-Analysis(pt) or Randomized Controlled Trial(pt)

Table adapted from *Users' Guides to the Medical Literature*[6].

> MeSH = Medical Subject Heading
> pt = Publication Type
> Explode = inclusion of all narrower MeSH

---

6   Guyatt G, Drummond R. *Users' Guides to the Medical Literature: Essentials of Evidence-Based Clinical Practice*. Chicago: American Medical Association, 2002.

Worked example: Ovid MEDLINE

What is the risk of type II diabetes for adults who are obese and take little exercise? Type of question: HARM

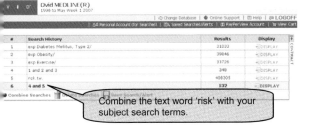

Combine the text word 'risk' with your subject search terms.

Clinical Queries

There are comprehensive, validated methodological search filters available for use developed by Haynes RB et al. These filters can be applied to your searches in Medline (using PubMed, Ovid or Dialog) – they are known as Clinical Queries.

The filters contain search terms (including publication types and free text words) designed to retrieve particular clinical study types. There are categories for etiology (harm), diagnosis, therapy and prognosis, corresponding to the four main types of clinical question.

To see details about the search strategies that make up these filters, go to the Clinical Queries filter table on the PubMed web page: www.ncbi.nlm.nih.gov/entrez/query/static/clinicaltable.html

Worked example: PubMed (www.pubmed.gov)

Recommend this site to a friend

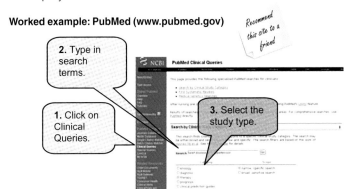

2. Type in search terms.

1. Click on Clinical Queries.

3. Select the study type.

Worked example: Ovid MEDLINE and Dialog MEDLINE

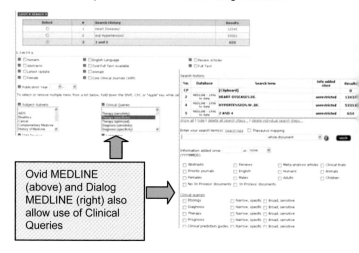

Ovid MEDLINE (above) and Dialog MEDLINE (right) also allow use of Clinical Queries

Sensitivity versus specificity

The terms 'sensitivity' and 'specificity' each have two meanings in evidence-based healthcare – one for statistics and one for searching. The application of sensitivity and specificity filters when searching is another way of refining your search.

The use of these terms in statistics refers to the accuracy of a diagnostic test. In the case of statistics, 'sensitivity' refers to how good a test is at correctly identifying people who have the disease, whereas 'specificity' is more concerned with how good the test is at correctly identifying people who are well.[7] Ideally, they should both be 100%, but this is rarely the case. In the context of searching, the terms again apply to accuracy, but this time in terms of number of results retrieved.

---

7   Loong TW. Understanding sensitivity and specificity with the right side of the brain. Br Med J 2003;327:716–719 (http://www.bmj.com/cgi/content/full/327/7417/716).

You can perform a *sensitive* (broad) or a *specific* (narrow) search when using Clinical Queries.

> Sensitivity = high recall, low precision (i.e. retrieves more of the relevant articles, but at the expense of picking up more unwanted stuff)
>
> Specificity = lower recall, higher precision (i.e. more of the articles retrieved will be relevant (proportionally), but some of the relevant stuff may be missed)

For example, a sensitive search may pick up 200 of the 225 relevant articles on your topic in Medline, but will also retrieve 500 irrelevant articles (total recall of 700). A specific search may pick up only 100 of the relevant 225 articles in Medline, but will only retrieve 50 irrelevant articles (total recall of 150).

When using Clinical Queries, a sensitive search will retrieve a greater number of the available articles of relevant study design, but will also pick up many unwanted articles. Proportionally, more of the articles retrieved in a specific search will be of a relevant study design, but some available relevant articles will be missed.

However, Clinical Queries only searches the PubMed content. There are other clinical databases where you will find relevant research, and although there is some overlap, there will also be new content on these databases. You can read more about other clinical databases in Chapter 3: Sources of clinical information: an overview.

Some of these databases will also have in-built filters, but for those that do not, you will have to construct your own filters. This is easily done, as many filters are widely available on the Internet. Just type in the terms that they have used, or as near to the terms as possible, and save the search so that you can return to it. Here are some resources:

⇒ Clinical Queries filters
   www.ncbi.nlm.nih.gov/entrez/query/static/clinicaltable.html
⇒ Centre for Reviews and Dissemination
   www.york.ac.uk/inst/crd/search.htm
⇒ Scottish Intercollegiate Guidelines Network
   www.sign.ac.uk/methodology/filters.html

For more help, contact your local medical librarian or use the help pages on the databases that you are using.

How do I do know whether to conduct a specific or sensitive search?

This depends on factors such as how much time you have, the reason you are doing the search and how much evidence there is on your topic. Choosing to conduct a sensitive search will mean the search will be more inclusive – you are less likely to miss something relevant, but you will need more time to look through the results for relevance.

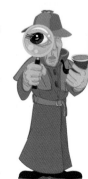

Conversely, the results from a specific search will take less time to look through and many will be relevant, but you have to accept that you won't have retrieved all the relevant articles – you may wish to use a specific search to find quickly articles of appropriate study design for use in immediate patient care.

Systematic reviews

There are several important databases containing systematic reviews, including the Cochrane Library and the Database of Abstracts of Reviews of Effectiveness (DARE) (see Chapter 3: Sources of clinical information: an overview). However, Medline also indexes systematic reviews and meta-analyses, and these can be quickly found by using the Find Systematic Reviews search box in PubMed Clinical Queries (www.pubmed.gov).

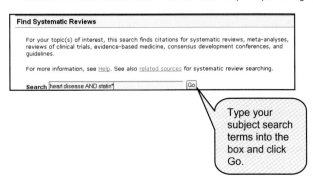

Find Systematic Reviews

For your topic(s) of interest, this search finds citations for systematic reviews, meta-analyses, reviews of clinical trials, evidence-based medicine, consensus development conferences, and guidelines.

For more information, see Help. See also related sources for systematic review searching.

Search heart disease AND statin*   Go

Type your subject search terms into the box and click Go.

9. Searching specific healthcare databases

Whichever resource you choose to search, the principles remain the same:

- Define a clear, answerable question before beginning your search – Chapter 5.
- Make a list of terms and synonyms – Chapter 6.
- Choose appropriate resources - Chapters 3 and 4.
- If unfamiliar with the information source, use the help pages/search tips of that resource – Chapter 9 and Appendix 1.
- Use truncation and/or wildcards where appropriate – Chapters 6 and 8.
- Combine with Boolean operators – Chapter 6.
- Use a combination of MeSH and free text searching – Chapter 7.

All searchable resources will have help sheets and/or tutorials available. Make use of these, and if you still need help, contact your local librarian.

There are five main providers of healthcare databases:
1. *Thomson Dialog* – access to AMED, British Nursing Index, EMBASE, MEDLINE and PsycInfo.
2. *EBSCO* – access to CINAHL.
3. *National Library of Medicine* – access to a free version of MEDLINE, known as PubMed.
4. *Ovid Wolters Kluwer* – access to AMED, British Nursing Index, EMBASE, MEDLINE and PsycInfo.
5. *Cochrane Library* – access to systematic reviews on treatments and research methodology, and database of systematic reviews.

Greater detail about healthcare databases can be found in Chapter 3: Sources of clinical information: an overview. Further hints and tips on searching can be found in Chapter 7: Free text versus thesaurus, and below.

This chapter will demonstrate the functionality of Medline Dialog, Medline Ovid, PubMed, CINAHL EBSCO and Cochrane Library to highlight the differences between software providers. At the end of Chapter 6 there is a summary table detailing which forms each software provider uses for truncation, wildcards, and Boolean operators.

To demonstrate how to perform a search on these databases, we will use the same scenario below for all five interfaces. Note that we have included numbers of hits retrieved for example purposes, but these depend on the date of the search, how often the interface is updated and features such as automatic MeSH mapping – these will differ between interface and repeats of the same search.

Scenario: A 1-year-old girl is admitted to the paediatrics department with bronchiolitis, where she is given a course of steroids. This prompts the doctor on duty to find out whether there is any evidence that corticosteroids lead to fewer hospital stays or improved recovery where bronchiolitis is concerned.

Focused question: Among young children with bronchiolitis, does treatment with corticosteroids lead to fewer hospital stays or improved recovery?

Patient/Problem	Intervention	Comparison	Outcome
Bronchiolitis	Corticosteroids OR Steroids	None	Stays OR Hospitalization OR Improvement OR Recovery

Type of question: intervention/treatment

Best feasible study design: systematic review or randomized controlled trial

---

Medline

Medline is the major bibliographic database for biomedical literature, and covers subjects such as medicine, dentistry, nursing and allied health. The database contains citations and abstracts from biomedical journals published in the USA, UK and many other countries.

Medline is provided electronically by a variety of publishers, three of which we cover in this chapter:
- PubMed (freely available)
- Ovid (subscription)
- Dialog (subscription)

PubMed (www.pubmed.gov)
PubMed is provided by the National Library of Medicine (USA) and includes all the citations from MEDLINE. It is freely available to anyone with an Internet connection.

Search process
Can I just type *bronchiolitis AND steroids* into the main search box?
Yes, but this retrieves 472 hits – do you want to look at them all?

PubMed tries automatically to map words to appropriate MeSH – if this is possible, both the free text and the MeSH will be included in the search. For more details, see the section on 'Ovid Medline'.

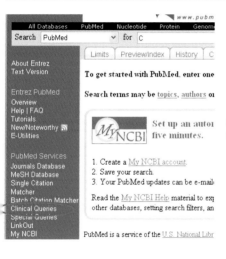

1. Try using the *Find Systematic Reviews* search box in Clinical Queries

Click on the Clinical Queries link to start.

Enter terms:

ind Systematic Reviews

For your topic(s) of interest, this search finds citations for systematic reviews, meta-analyses, reviews of clinical trials, evidence-based medicine, consensus development conferences, and guidelines.

For more information, see Help. See also related sources for systematic review searching.

Search bronchiolitis AND steroids   Go

> Note: when using the filters on Clinical Queries, you are restricting your PubMed search quite considerably, so begin by using only the key terms, and by making your search quite broad (i.e. do not combine too many search terms together with 'AND'). If you make your search too narrow when using Clinical Queries you will retrieve very little. You can always narrow the search later if necessary.

This search retrieved 12 hits, including a relevant systematic review published in 2004:

Davison C et al. Efficacy of interventions for bronchiolitis in critically ill infants: a systematic review and meta-analysis. Pediatr Crit Care Med. 2004 Sep;5(5):482–9.

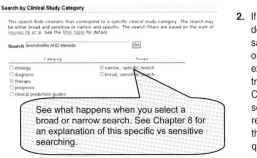

Search by Clinical Study Category

This search finds citations that correspond to a specific clinical study category. The search may be either broad and sensitive or narrow and specific. The search filters are based on the work of Haynes RB et al. See the filter table for details.

Search [bronchiolitis AND steroids] [Go]

Category	Scope
○ etiology	● narrow, specific search
○ diagnosis	○ broad, sensitive search
● therapy	
○ prognosis	
○ clinical prediction guides	

See what happens when you select a broad or narrow search. See Chapter 8 for an explanation of this specific vs sensitive searching.

2. If the above search does not yield satisfactory results, or you wish to expand the search, try using the main Clinical Queries search box, and restricting to therapy as type of question.

This search retrieved 43 hits (narrow search), including a relevant randomized controlled trial:

Zhang L et al. Long and short-term effect of prednisolone in hospitalized infants with acute bronchiolitis. J Paediatr Child Health. 2003 Sep-Oct;39(7):548–51.

What if using Clinical Queries has not retrieved any results that help me to answer my question?

You must expand your search to the whole of PubMed, and use the search techniques we learnt in Chapter 7: Free text versus thesaurus.

> Tip: Return to the main PubMed search screen by clicking the PubMed logo at the top of the screen, or the PubMed link on the top (black) index bar.

3. Include a free text term and a Medical Subject Heading (MeSH) for each relevant PICO term whenever possible.

Free text

Think of all the alternative spellings for free text, and make use of truncation (* symbol on PubMed) to expand word endings.

For example:

hospitalisation OR hospitalization	Includes UK and US spellings
corticosteroid*	Finds *corticosteroid* (singular) and *corticosteroids* (plural).
improv*	Finds *improve, improves, improved, improving,* etc.

Note: Be careful not to truncate too near the beginning of words, because you will retrieve too many different words. For example, imp* will find not only the above words but also everything else beginning with imp. You will also find that if there are too many word endings, a message will appear stating 'Wildcard search for 'imp*' used only the first 600 variations. Lengthen the root word to search for all endings'.

MeSH

The following example shows how to find the MeSH term for corticosteroids.

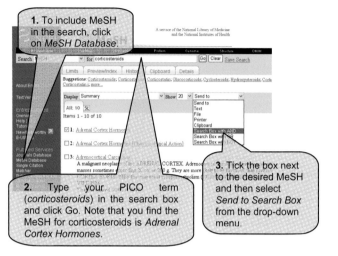

1. To include MeSH in the search, click on *MeSH Database*.

2. Type your PICO term (*corticosteroids*) in the search box and click Go. Note that you find the MeSH for corticosteroids is *Adrenal Cortex Hormones*.

3. Tick the box next to the desired MeSH and then select *Send to Search Box* from the drop-down menu.

Finally, click on the *Search PubMed* button to perform the MeSH search.

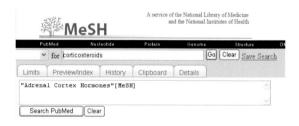

Relevant citations in MEDLINE may be indexed with the MeSH *Adrenal Cortex Hormones*, or contain the free text word *corticosteroids* in the title or abstract, or both. This particular example demonstrates the importance of using both MeSH and free text in your search, to allow for use of either term in a citation.

Combining search terms
Free text and MeSH can be combined using Boolean logic (AND, OR).

Chapter 6: Building a search strategy

Remember:
Combine similar concepts with OR to expand the search ('OR means more').
Combine different concepts with AND to narrow the search

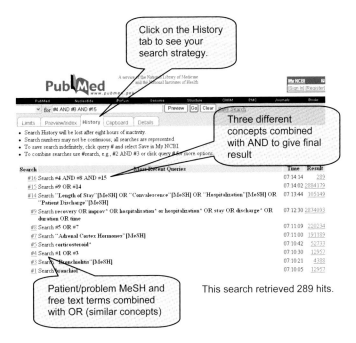

Click on the History tab to see your search strategy.

Three different concepts combined with AND to give final result

Patient/problem MeSH and free text terms combined with OR (similar concepts)

This search retrieved 289 hits.

An example of a finished search strategy is shown above. Each line is numbered, for example #1 – these line numbers can be used when combining searches.

Viewing the results

Click on the number of hits next to the line you want to view, that is, 289 above. The title and author details will be displayed in batches of 20 – to view more (or less) records on one page, select a number from the Show drop-down menu.

To see the abstract for an individual article, click on the abstract symbol next to the record. If the abstract symbol has a green band at the top, this means that a free full-text version is available. Other articles have full-text versions available but they require a subscription, either individually or via your institution.

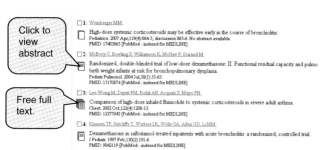

To see abstracts of *all* displayed articles, choose *Abstract* (or *Citation*) from the *Display* drop-down menu. You can also sort the records by publication date, author or journal title by using the *Sort* menu.

Clipboard

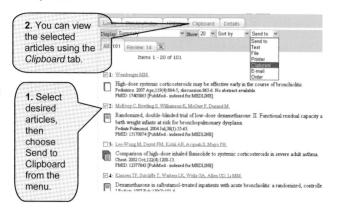

Saving, printing or emailing records

Using the *Send to* drop-down menu you can choose to *Print*, save to *File* or *Email* your results.

> If you wish to import citations from PubMed into a Citation Manager database, you will need to select *Send to File*. This allows you to save your citations as a text file, which can be imported into a Citation Manager (see Chapter 11: Saving/recording citations for future use). There is currently no direct export facility available in PubMed. **Before you do this**, use the Display menu to change the format of your records to MEDLINE. Then when you Send to File, the records will be saved in a format that can be recognized by citation managers.

Related Article feature

Another way to find potentially relevant articles is to use the Related Article feature.

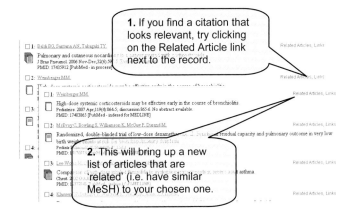

1. If you find a citation that looks relevant, try clicking on the Related Article link next to the record.

2. This will bring up a new list of articles that are 'related' (i.e. have similar MeSH) to your chosen one.

MEDLINE Dialog (http://www.dialog.com/)

Thomson Dialog provides an interface on the World Wide Web for searching the MEDLINE database. It is a subscription service, often available via libraries, universities or hospitals.

Search process

Can I just type *bronchiolitis AND steroids* into the main search box?
Yes, but this retrieves 230 hits – do you want to look at them all?

Few of the citations on the beginning pages look particularly relevant to the question.

1. Try using Clinical Queries, and restricting to *Therapy* as type of question. On the main search page, type *bronchiolitis AND steroids*, then click the Search button. After the search has been performed, click on *Clinical Queries*, then select the type of question.

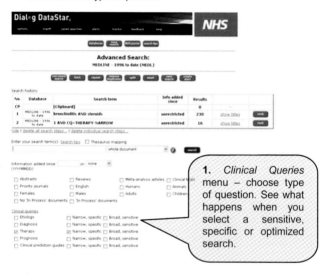

> 1. *Clinical Queries* menu – choose type of question. See what happens when you select a sensitive, specific or optimized search.

This search retrieved 16 hits (using the specific search), including a relevant randomized controlled trial:

Plint AC et al. Practice variation among pediatric emergency departments in the treatment of bronchiolitis. Academic Emergency Medicine 2004;11(4):353–360

Why was the randomized trial (Zhang et al.) retrieved from PubMed Clinical Queries (Therapy question, narrow) not found using the above same search in Dialog MEDLINE?

PubMed tries to map all words automatically to appropriate MeSH – if this is possible, both the free text and the MeSH will be included in the search. PubMed will always default to *Explode* the MeSH.

Explode = inclusion of all narrower MeSH. Many MeSH are subdivided into further headings – if you wish to include all these narrower subject headings, you must *Explode* the MeSH. Exploding is a way of broadening your search.

e.g.   *Steroids*

Androstanes
Bile Acids and Salts
Cardanolides
Cholanes
… etc.

Exploding *Steroids* will also search for citations with any of the narrower subject headings above.

Dialog will also try automatically to map to appropriate MeSH, but Dialog does NOT *Explode* MeSH unless requested. So PubMed includes the MeSH *Steroids and all narrower subject headings*, but Dialog MEDLINE only includes the MeSH *Steroids*. This accounts for the difference in the number of hits obtained, and why the randomized trial found in PubMed is not retrieved using (apparently) the same search in Dialog.

To make sure you include both *Exploded* MeSH and free text when using Dialog MEDLINE, search each term separately – for example, type *bronchiolitis* into the search box, make sure the *Map Term to Subject Heading* box is selected, and click the Search button. Dialog will then display a list of possible MeSH, giving you the option to *Explode*, and to include the free text word, as overleaf.

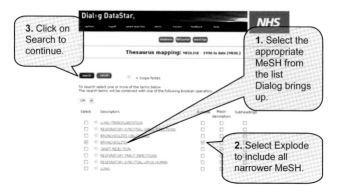

Combine the free text and the thesaurus term using OR.
Repeat for the search term *steroids*. Finally combine the two different search concepts using AND.

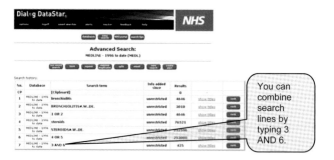

2. Repeating the *Clinical Queries* search on *Therapy* (specific) using the above search, now retrieves the same 43 hits obtained from PubMed Clinical Queries (including the randomized trial by *Zhang L et al*).

What if using Clinical Queries has not retrieved any results that help me to answer my question?

You can broaden your search using the search techniques we learnt in Chapter 7.

Chapter 7: Free text versus thesaurus

3. Include a free text term and a Medical Subject Heading (MeSH) for each relevant PICO term whenever possible.

Free text
Think of all the alternative spellings for free text, and make use of truncation ($ symbol on Dialog) to expand word endings.

For example:

hospitalisation OR hospitalization	Includes UK and US spellings
corticosteroid$	Finds *corticosteroid* (singular) *and* *corticosteroids* (plural)
improv$	Finds *improve, improves, improved, improving,* etc.

The truncation symbol on Dialog is $. It is advisable to limit the truncation by putting a number after the $ sign. For example, nurs$3 will search for nurse, nurses, nursing, whereas doctor$1 will search for doctor or doctors. Make sure you turn off the thesaurus mapping option when you search using truncation.

MeSH
Use the *Map Term to Subject Heading* box for each PICO term, as in the Clinical Queries example above.

Combining search terms
Free text and MeSH can be combined using Boolean logic (AND, OR). Combine similar concepts with OR, different concepts with AND. More information about this is given in Chapter 6: Building a search strategy.

An example of a finished search strategy is shown overleaf. Each line is numbered – these line numbers can be used when combining searches. Alternatively you can combine by clicking on Combine Searches, and selecting the appropriate searches and Boolean terms.

Advanced Search:
MEDLINE - 1996 to date (MEDL)

Search history:

No.	Database	Search term	Info added since	Results		
CP		[Clipboard]		0		
1	MEDLINE - 1996 to date	bronchiolitis	unrestricted	4646	show titles	rank
2	MEDLINE - 1996 to date	BRONCHIOLITIS#.W..DE.	unrestricted	3018	show titles	rank
3	MEDLINE - 1996 to date	1 OR 2	unrestricted	4646	show titles	rank
4	MEDLINE - 1996 to date	steroids	unrestricted	76521	show titles	rank
5	MEDLINE - 1996 to date	STEROIDS#.W..DE.	unrestricted	212596	show titles	rank
6	MEDLINE - 1996 to date	4 OR 5	unrestricted	253000	show titles	rank
7	MEDLINE - 1996 to date	3 AND 6	unrestricted	425	show titles	rank
8	MEDLINE - 1996 to date	recovery	unrestricted	141371	show titles	rank
9	MEDLINE - 1996 to date	length ADJ of ADJ stay	unrestricted	23893	show titles	rank
10	MEDLINE - 1996 to date	LENGTH-OF-STAY#.DE.	unrestricted	23893	show titles	rank
11	MEDLINE - 1996 to date	improv$4	unrestricted	473965	show titles	rank
12	MEDLINE - 1996 to date	discharge$4	unrestricted	72271	show titles	rank
13	MEDLINE - 1996 to date	convalescence	unrestricted	2469	show titles	rank
14	MEDLINE - 1996 to date	CONVALESCENCE#.W..DE.	unrestricted	1038	show titles	rank
15	MEDLINE - 1996 to date	hospitalisation	unrestricted	55017	show titles	rank
16	MEDLINE - 1996 to date	HOSPITALIZATION#.W..DE.	unrestricted	60035	show titles	rank
17	MEDLINE - 1996 to date	8 OR 9 OR 10 OR 11 OR 12 OR 13 OR 14 OR 15 OR 16	unrestricted	715291	show titles	rank
18	MEDLINE - 1996 to date	7 AND 17	unrestricted	130	show titles	rank

Viewing the results

Click on the *Show Titles* link next to the line you want to view. The title and author details will be displayed in batches of 10 – to view more (or less) records on one page, click on *Customize Display* and change the citations per page. You can also choose to see abstracts of **all** displayed articles from this page. To see the abstract for an individual article, click on the *Link to abstract/database record* link next to the record. If there is a *Full Text* link next to the record, this means that a free full-text version is available (usually via your institution).

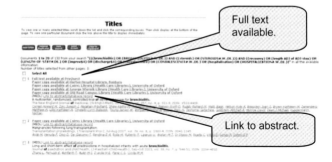

Full text available.

Link to abstract.

Displaying, saving, printing or emailing records

Using the *Results Manager* at the bottom of the page you can choose to *Display, Print, Email* or *Save* your results. You can choose to Save all records or just a selection.

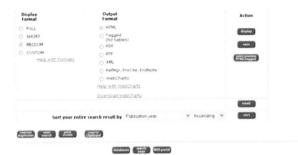

If you wish to import citations *directly* from Dialog MEDLINE into a Citation Manager database (see Chapter 11: Saving/recording citations for future use), you will need to select *RefMgr, ProCite EndNote*, and *Save* from the Results Manager.

You can sort your results by choosing an option from the drop-down menu. Dialog automatically sorts by publication year.

WebCharts

Dialog has its own Citation Manager, which is very simple to download and use. It is called WebCharts and is very similar to the spreadsheets in Microsoft Excel.

Saving searches

Click on the Save Search button, and this will take you to a new screen, where you can save your search, enabling you to rerun searches at a later date. You can also edit searches that you have run previously, in case you want to add additional terms.

Alerts

The Alerts function allows you to receive updates related to your search strategy, so that each time an article matching your search criteria is added to the database, an email is sent to you, notifying you of the new addition. You can also receive these updates via RSS feeds, which send information to an aggregator of your choice. This enables you to get the latest evidence in your field, without having to rerun the search regularly.

MEDLINE Ovid (http://www.ovid.com/)

Ovid Technologies (part of Wolters Kluwer Health) provides an interface on the World Wide Web for searching the MEDLINE database. It is a subscription service, often available via libraries, universities or hospitals.

Search process

Can I just type *bronchiolitis AND steroids* into the main search box?
Yes, but this retrieves 173 hits – do you want to look at them all?

Few of the citations on the beginning pages look particularly relevant to the question.

1. Try using Clinical Queries, and restricting to *Therapy* as type of question. On the main search page, type *bronchiolitis AND steroids*, then click the Search button. After the search has been performed, click on *More Limits*. Then select the type of question, as below.

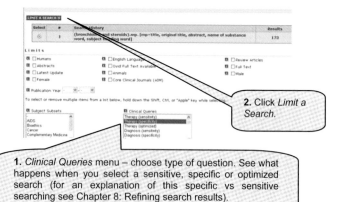

2. Click *Limit a Search.*

1. *Clinical Queries* menu – choose type of question. See what happens when you select a sensitive, specific or optimized search (for an explanation of this specific vs sensitive searching see Chapter 8: Refining search results).

This search retrieved 18 hits (using the specific search), including a relevant randomized controlled trial:

Wong JY et al. No objective benefit from steroids inhaled via a spacer in infants recovering from bronchiolitis. European Respiratory Journal 2000 Feb;15(2):388–94.

Why was the randomized trial (Zhang et al.) retrieved from PubMed Clinical Queries (Therapy question, narrow) not found using the above same search in Ovid MEDLINE?

PubMed tries to map all words automatically to appropriate MeSH – if this is possible, both the free text and the MeSH will be included in the search. PubMed will always default to *Explode* the MeSH. Ovid will also try to map automatically to appropriate MeSH, but Ovid does NOT *Explode* MeSH unless requested. See section on MEDLINE Dialog earlier in the chapter for more details.

To make sure you include both *Exploded* MeSH and free text when using Ovid MEDLINE, search each term separately. For example, type *bronchiolitis* into the search box, make sure the *Map Term to Subject Heading* box is selected, and click the Search button. Ovid will then display a list of possible MeSH, giving you the option to *Explode*, and to include the free text word, as below.

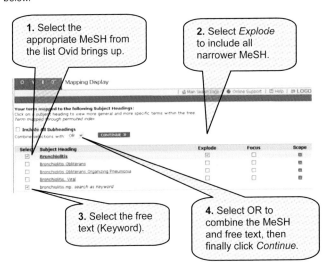

2. Repeat for the search term *steroids*. Finally combine the two different search concepts using AND.

#	Search History	Results	Display
1	bronchiolitis.mp. or exp Bronchiolitis/	6420	+ DISPLAY
2	steroids.mp. or exp Steroids/	599938	+ DISPLAY
3	1 and 2	471	+ DISPLAY

🔗 Combine Searches 🗑 Delete Searches 💾 Save Search/Alert

> You can combine search lines by typing 1 AND 2.

Repeating the *Clinical Queries* search on *Therapy* (specific) using the above search, now retrieves the same 43 hits obtained from PubMed Clinical Queries (including the randomized trial by *Zhang L et al*).

What if using Clinical Queries has not retrieved any results that help me to answer my question?

You can broaden your search using the search techniques we learnt in Chapter 7.

> Chapter 7: Free text versus thesaurus

3. Include a free text term and a Medical Subject Heading (MeSH) for each relevant PICO term whenever possible.

Free text
Think of all the alternative spellings for free text, and make use of truncation ($ symbol on Ovid) to expand word endings.

For example:

hospitalisation OR hospitalization	Includes UK and US spellings
corticosteroid$	Finds *corticosteroid* (singular) *and corticosteroids* (plural)
improv$	Finds *improve, improves, improved, improving* etc.

The truncation symbol on Ovid is $. Note that automatic MeSH mapping does NOT work when truncation is used.

MeSH
Use the *Map Term to Subject Heading* box for each PICO term, as in the Clinical Queries example above.

Combining search terms
Free text and MeSH can be combined using Boolean logic (AND, OR). Combine similar concepts with OR, different concepts with AND. You will find more about this concept in Chapter 6.

> Chapter 6: Building a search strategy

An example of a finished search strategy is shown below. Each line is numbered – these line numbers can be used when combining searches. Alternatively you can combine by clicking on Combine Searches, and selecting the appropriate searches and Boolean terms.

#	Search History	Results
1	bronchiolitis.mp. or exp Bronchiolitis/	6420
2	corticosteroids.mp. or exp Adrenal Cortex Hormones/	282210
3	recovery.mp.	195494
4	exp "Length of Stay"/ or stay.mp.	69559
5	improv$.mp. [mp=title, original title, abstract, name of substance word, subject heading word]	707348
6	discharge$.mp. [mp=title, original title, abstract, name of substance word, subject heading word]	102098
7	convalescence.mp. or exp Convalescence/	5176
8	exp Hospitalization/ or hospitalisation.mp.	106233
9	hospitalization.mp.	81060
10	3 or 4 or 5 or 6 or 7 or 8 or 9	1077896
11	1 and 2 and 10	210

👀 Combine Searches 🗑 Delete Searches 🔖 Save Search/Alert

Viewing the results
Click on the *Display* link next to the line you want to view. The title and author details will be displayed in batches of 10 – to view more (or less) records on one page, click on *Customize Display* and change the citations per page. You can also choose to see abstracts of **all** displayed articles from this page.

To see the abstract for an individual article, click on the *Abstract* link next to the record. If there is a *Full Text* link next to the record, this means that a free full-text version is available (usually via your institution). Other articles may have the full text available, but they require a subscription.

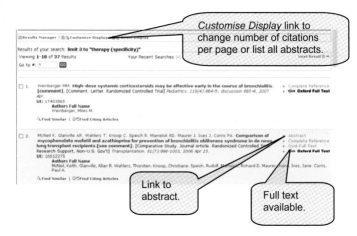

Customise Display link to change number of citations per page or list all abstracts.

Link to abstract.

Full text available.

Saving, printing or emailing records

Using the *Results Manager* at the bottom of the page you can choose to *Print*, *Email* or *Save* your results. You can choose to Save all records or just a selection.

> If you wish to import citations *directly* from Ovid MEDLINE into a Citation Manager database (see Chapter 11: Saving/recording citations for future use), you will need to select *Direct Export*, and *Save* from the Results Manager.

Find similar articles

Another way to find potentially relevant articles is to use the *Find Similar* feature (like the Related Article feature on PubMed). However, this feature on Ovid is not as extensive as on PubMed, where many Related Articles are displayed.

EBSCO provides an interface on the World Wide Web for searching the CINAHL database. CINAHL provides indexing for 3123 journals from the fields of nursing and allied health, with indexing back to 1937. It is a subscription service, often available via libraries, universities or hospitals.

Search process

There are two ways of searching CINAHL, the basic search and the advanced search. The difference is that with Advanced Search, you can see your search history, save it and set up alerts. Advanced Search will, therefore, give you more functionality.

Can I just type *asthma AND nurses* into the main search box?
Yes, but this retrieves 486 hits – do you want to look at them all?

Few of the citations on the beginning pages look particularly relevant to the question.

Free text

Think of all the alternative spellings for free text, and make use of truncation to expand word endings. The truncation symbol on EBSCO is *.

For example:

asthma OR respiratory disorder	Includes variations in terminology
*nurse**	Finds *nurse* (singular) *and nurses* (plural)
*nurs**	Finds *nurse, nurses, nursing,* etc.

MeSH/thesaurus

CINAHL has a thesaurus too, a version of MeSH called 'CINAHL Headings'.

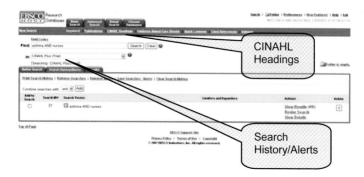

Click on CINAHL Headings, type in your first term and click on Browse. A list of terms will be displayed. Choose the most relevant term, tick the Explode box, and click on Search Database.

You can combine more than one term, but it is more useful to search for each term individually, so that you can change your combinations in the search history. You do also have the option to incorporate the Free Text term into your search strategy.

There is an option to select Major Concept, which asks the database to find only papers where the subject heading is the main focus of the article. It is best to avoid this option because it can limit your search too much and you may miss out on some key papers.

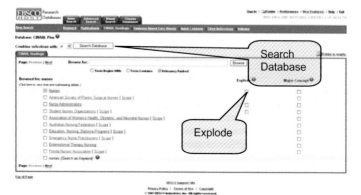

If you want to see more about what the term covers, click on the link and you will be taken to the following screen, where you can also select headings (although use these with care because they can limit the search too much).

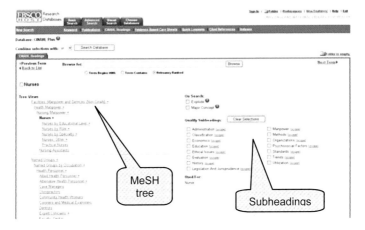

Repeat this step using 'CINAHL Headings' with the other terms in your search strategy.

Combining search terms

Free text and MeSH can be combined using Boolean logic (AND, OR). Combine similar concepts with OR, different concepts with AND. This concept is discussed more fully in Chapter 6: Building a search strategy.

Once you have all your search terms, click on Search History/Alerts and combine the searches as appropriate.

An example of a finished search strategy is shown below. Each line is numbered (e.g. S1, S2) – these line numbers can be used when combining searches. Alternatively you can combine by ticking the appropriate boxes, choosing the combination term, clicking on Add, and then on Search.

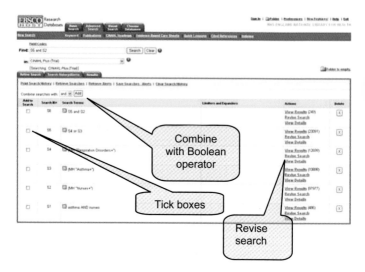

Limiting searches

In the Search History, on the right of the screen, there is an option to 'Revise Search'. If you click on this you will be taken to another screen, where you can set your limits.

Viewing the results

After clicking on Search, all the results are automatically displayed. You then have options to view by different publication types, or filtered by subject area. To save any of the items, you just need to add them to the folder on the right of the screen. To save them for future use, you need to be logged in. Click on the title to see the abstract. If full text is available, the links are clearly visible below the citation.

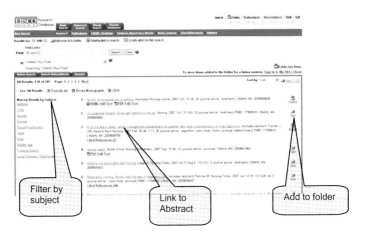

Filter by subject

Link to Abstract

Add to folder

Saving, printing or emailing records

When you are ready to print out, email, save or export to citation manager software, click on the folder at the top of the screen, and choose the appropriate option. This is also where searches and alerts will be saved.

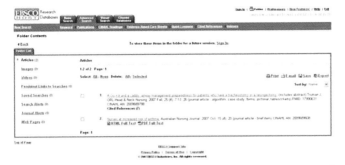

If you wish to import citations *directly* from EBSCO CINAHL into a Citation Manager database (see Chapter 11: Saving/recording citations for future use), you will need to select Export and choose the relevant software.

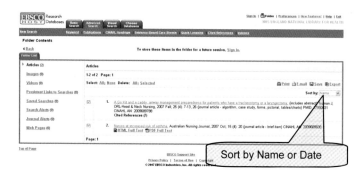

You can sort your results by choosing an option from the drop-down menu. EBSCO automatically sorts by title.

Saving searches
Return to the Search History, and click on the Save Searches/Alerts option. Here you will be able to log in and save your searches so that you can come back to them and re-run them should you need to.

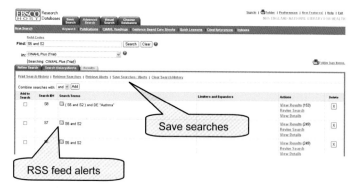

Alerts
The alerts function allows you to receive updates related to your search strategy, so that each time an article matching your search criteria is added to the database, an email is sent to you, notifying you of the new addition. You can also receive these updates via RSS feeds, which send information to an aggregator of your choice. This enables you to get the latest evidence

in your field, without having to re-run the search regularly. Just click on the orange button next to the search you are interested in, and cut and paste the 'syndication feed' into your chosen aggregator.

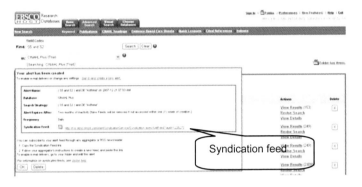

Syndication feed

What are RSS feeds?

RSS feeds are a way of receiving information and keeping up-to-date. Many websites are providing RSS feeds, and you can recognize them with symbols similar to this one or with RSS or XML in white with an orange background. To read the feeds you need to set up a page on a news reader or an aggregator, such as Bloglines (www.bloglines.com). This page will collect all of your RSS feeds. It sounds complicated, but once the page is set up you don't need to do anything else. Every time your favourite websites are updated, they will automatically send details to your news reader. This means that instead of visiting lots of websites to see if there is any new content, you can just go to one and see all the updates. It also means that your email box will not be overflowing with emails.

RSS feeds are particularly useful for journal content pages and search results, so that each time new research is added to the database that fits with your search criteria, you will automatically be alerted to this. A useful tutorial on RSS is available from Common Craft (www.commoncraft.com). The video, called 'RSS in Plain English', is available at: http://www.commoncraft.com/rss_plain_english.

Cochrane Library (www.thecochranelibrary.com)

The Cochrane Library is a collection of databases that contain high-quality, independent evidence to inform healthcare decision-making. Cochrane Reviews represent the highest level of evidence on which to base clinical treatment decisions. There are 51 Cochrane Review groups providing systematic reviews. In addition to these reviews, there are systematic reviews from other providers, technology assessments, economic evaluations and individual clinical trials. There are different levels of access, and more information can be found here:

www3.interscience.wiley.com/cgi-bin/mrwhome/106568753/
AccessCochraneLibrary.html

!	**NOTE!**
	For clinical searches, the Cochrane Library is a good place to start. However, bear in mind that you will retrieve less hits than other healthcare databases, because the content is mainly systematic reviews and randomized controlled trials. There are currently only 5053 records in the Cochrane Library, compared with over 17 million citations in PubMed!

Search process

There are three ways of searching the Cochrane Library: the basic search, the advanced search and the MeSH search. The advanced search allows you to combine terms and apply limits. The MeSH search gives you access to the thesaurus.

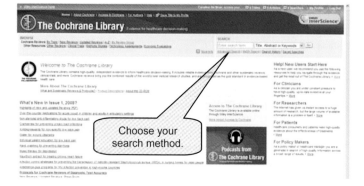

Choose your search method.

Can I just type *asthma AND nurses* into the main search box?
Yes, but this retrieves only 2 hits, neither of which looks useful.

You will retrieve more relevant results by using the Advanced search or the MeSH search.

Advanced search

Think of all the alternative spellings for free text, and make use of truncation to expand word endings. The truncation symbol in the Cochrane Library is *.

For example:

asthma OR respiratory disorder	Includes variations in terminology
nurse*	Finds *nurse* (singular) *and nurses* (plural)
nurs*	Finds *nurse, nurses, nursing,* etc.

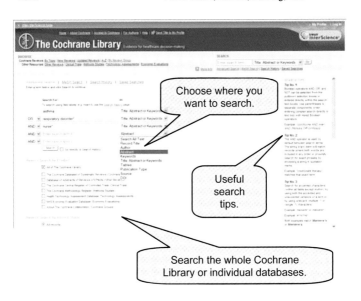

Choose where you want to search.

Useful search tips.

Search the whole Cochrane Library or individual databases.

MeSH

The Cochrane Library has a thesaurus, a version of MeSH called 'MeSH Search'. When you access this search, you have the option to enter your term and go straight to the MeSH Trees. You can also browse the thesaurus, by entering your term and clicking on Thesaurus, and if you want to check a definition, just enter your term and click on Definition.

Click on MeSH Search, type in your first term and click on Go to MeSH Trees. A list of terms, including the one you have entered, will be displayed. The database will automatically EXPLODE the term, unless you select a tree and/or click on Search this term only. Click on View Results. You have the option to 'Go directly to Search History', which is useful if you want to combine terms.

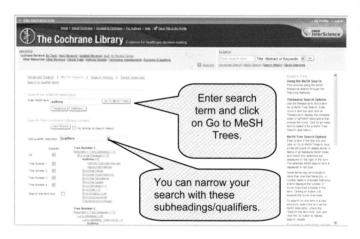

There is an option to add Qualifiers/Subheadings, but this can narrow the search considerably and you may miss out on some important records.

On the right-hand side of the screen there are useful search tips.

Repeat this process using MeSH Search with the other terms in your search strategy.

Combining search terms

All searches, whether performed as a basic Search, Advanced Search or MeSH Search, are automatically stored in the Search History. From there, you can combine them using Boolean logic (AND, OR). Combine similar concepts with OR, different concepts with AND. This process is discussed more fully in Chapter 6: Building a search strategy.

Once you have all your search terms, click on Search History and combine the searches as appropriate.

An example of a finished search strategy is shown below. Each line is numbered (e.g. #1, #2) – these line numbers should be used when combining searches.

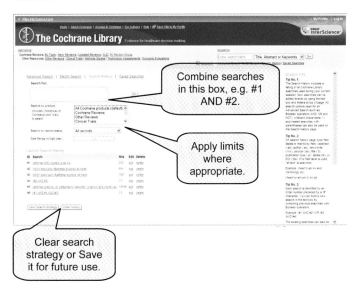

Limiting searches

In the Search History, below the search box, there are some options to limit by Product (e.g. type of publication), Record status (e.g. new, updated, or withdrawn) or by Date. There is no language limit because all Cochrane Reviews are available in a range of languages.

Viewing the results
In the Search History, you need to click on the search string to view the results. The results are organized by database:
- Cochrane Reviews
- Other Reviews
- Clinical Trials
- Methods Studies
- Technology Assessments
- Economic Evaluations
- Cochrane Groups

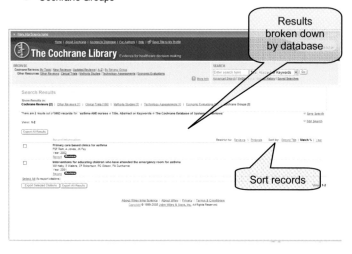

Results broken down by database

Sort records

Click on Record to access the full text, where this is available. In the Cochrane Reviews database, you can restrict the results to Reviews or Protocols. You can sort the results by Record Title, Match % or Year.

Saving, exporting or printing records
To save a search in a text format or export results to Endnote citation software, you need to register with Wiley InterScience. Registration is free to all Internet users.

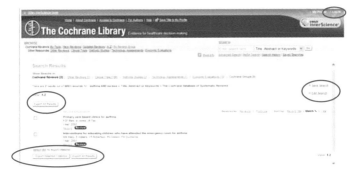

Click on the Log-in option at the top right-hand of the screen. Once logged onto the system, tick the records that you want to save or export, and click on the Export All or Selected option. The following screen will appear.

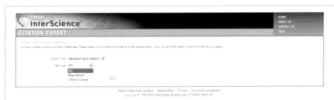

Make your choices and click on Go. The results can be saved or opened in the format of your choice.

Printing out can be done in two ways. Either follow the process of exporting the records and printing out the citation and abstract, or if you want to print the full text, you will need to go into each individual record. This is because the Cochrane Reviews can be very large documents and therefore need to be selected individually for printing. They are also on different databases and therefore have different formats for printing.

Saving searches

To save the search history, you need to register with Wiley InterScience. Registration is free to all Internet users. Click on the Log-in option at the top right-hand of the screen.

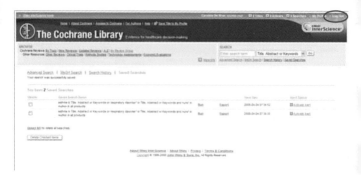

Alerts

The alerts function allows you to receive updates related to your search strategy, so that each time an article matching your search criteria is added to the database, an email is sent to you, notifying you of the new addition. This service is available to registered online users (see earlier in this section on registering with Wiley InterScience). The Alert function is displayed when you save your search. You are offered the option of Activating the alert for your saved search.

User guides

The Cochrane Library has help available, in a range of different languages: www3.interscience.wiley.com/cgi-bin/mrwhome/106568753/HELP_ Cochrane.html

10. *Citation pearl searching*

Sometimes when you have run your search, the results are not satisfactory. For example, out of 50 results you might only have found one that is relevant. So what do you do next?

Option 1
Give up and end up none the wiser.

Option 2
Investigate further and find the buried treasure!

Option 2 is **citation pearl searching**. It means taking the little that you do have and drawing more from it. There are a number of ways to do this.

Related items

Many databases and search engines now identify 'related items' or 'similar items' that could be what you are looking for. PubMed has 'Related Links':

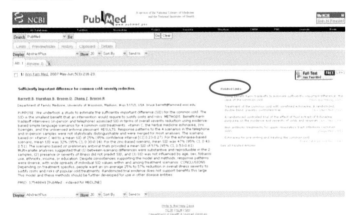

In the example above, a relevant article comparing the use of vitamin C and echinacea as a means of relieving the symptoms of the common cold was retrieved. The MeSH terms used were 'Common Cold' AND 'Ascorbic Acid' AND 'Echinacea'. Only eight results were found, of which this was the most appropriate. On the right of the screen, however, other papers are identified that did not appear in the original search but might be relevant.

Google offers 'Similar pages':

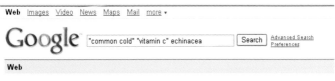

Author search

It is possible to search using an author's surname and initials to see what else they have written. Many journal websites already have links, such as 'Articles by [author name]' so that you can see if an author has written more papers on the same topic. On PubMed this is very easy because the author names are hyperlinked, so just clicking on the author's name takes you to other research by that author. This feature occurs in many healthcare databases.

Many papers will feature the author's contact details, so you can contact them directly to see if they have written (or indeed if they are writing) anything else on this topic or if they know of any other researchers who have written on the same topic.

Keywords

After performing a search, if you only find one good relevant reference, go into the full record and look at the **keywords**, **MeSH** terms, **descriptors**, etc. to see if they have been indexed using terms you have not included in your search. Sometimes, different terms are used in different countries. For example, the MEDLINE and CINAHL indexes use the term Allied Health Personnel, whereas EMBASE uses Paramedical Personnel for the same type of health profession. If all the terms are not included in the search, then you might miss out on key research.

In PubMed, if you change the Display to Citation or MEDLINE, the list of **MeSH** or **descriptors** headings will be shown:

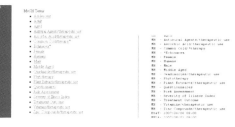

The *British Medical Journal*, along with other journals, offers a range of methods for citation pearl searching, including 'Articles by [author name]' on Google Scholar or PubMed, 'Related Articles' on the BMJ site (www.bmj. com) and 'Similar Articles in BMJ or PubMed':

References

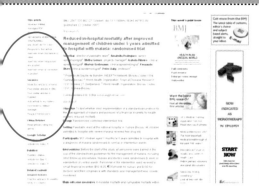

One final place to search for similar papers is in the list of references supplied by the author of the relevant article. Often this is a good place to look when searching for similar titles or for authors who are investigating the same topics. Particularly with online papers, the individual references may even hyperlink straight to the original papers.

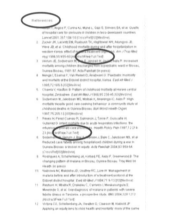

After the list of references, the *British Medical Journal* and some other journals display a list of 'Related Articles'. Following this, they identify papers that have cited the featured paper.

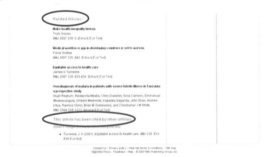

These types of journals offer three services:
1. Alert me when this article is cited
2. Alert me when responses are posted
3. Alert me when a correction is posted

This enables you to keep up to date with any changes in your field of research.

It is worth making a note of each stage of the citation pearl searching, in case you need to write up your literature review, but also so that you don't get lost!

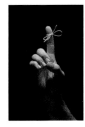

11. Saving/recording citations for future use

Scenario: *you perform a search using PubMed Clinical Queries, and feel pleased with yourself as you find a systematic review that helps you to treat a specific patient. Three months later, the same treatment question crops up again for a different patient, but you can't remember what the paper was or where you found it, so you have to do the search again.*

Does this sound familiar?

Below are two ways that you can record or save details about useful papers you find from your searches, so that you can retrieve them at a later date.

Logbooks

Use a paper notebook (or a word document) to jot down clinical questions when they arise, and if you have a chance to search for papers to answer some of them, write down the citation(s) and a summary of their results.

One example is the Centre for Evidence-Based Medicine (http://www.cebm.net) 'Asking Answerable Questions' logbook, which contains pages in a spiral-bound notebook – each page has space to write down your PICO question, the useful citation(s) you found and the clinical bottom line, as below.

PICO: *What is the risk of type II diabetes for adults who are obese and take little*

PICO: *In postmenopausal women, does oestrogen plus progestogen hormone therapy increase the risk of being diagnosed with breast cancer?*

Reference: *Chlebowski JAMA 2003;289:3243–53*

Clinical bottom line: *Women who received HT had a greater incidence of total and invasive breast cancer.*

All breast cancer hazard ratio 1.24 (1.02–1.50).
  Invasive breast cancer hazard ratio 1.24 (1.01–1.54).

Software

There are also software packages, or 'citation managers', that enable you to save details of useful citations.

> You may see software for saving, managing and publishing citations described as:
> *Citation managers*
> *Citation management software*
> *Bibliographic management software*
> *Bibliographic publishing tools*
> *Reference management software*

Citation managers allow you to export references directly from databases (e.g. Medline) or from some web pages (e.g. electronic journals like BMJ and JAMA). You can also add references manually, search, create a bibliography and 'cite while you write' (a facility to add citations to a document you are writing).

Specific citation managers include:
- ProCite: www.procite.com/
- Reference Manager: www.refman.com/
- EndNote: www.endnote.com/
- RefWorks: www.refworks.com/
- Biblioscape: www.biblioscape.com/ (free version)
- Biblioexpress: www.biblioscape.com/biblioexpress.htm

All of the above packages have similar features – most of them allow you to download a free trial before making a purchase.

The example below (from Ovid MEDLINE) shows the Direct Export of citations – clicking on Save will allow the export of selected MEDLINE citations to your citation manager.

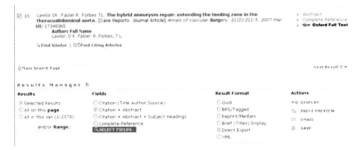

The example below shows a Reference Manager database after citations have been imported.

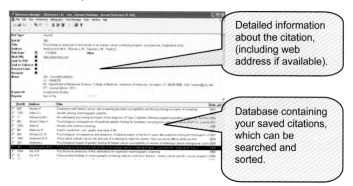

Detailed information about the citation, (including web address if available).

Database containing your saved citations, which can be searched and sorted.

Cite while you write

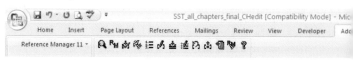

One of the neat things to learn is to cite while you write. It will save you loads of time in formatting your references and bibliography.

Cite While You Write gives you access to Reference Manager references and formatting commands with a submenu on Word's Tools menu.

12. Critical appraisal

The majority of content indexed in healthcare databases has not undergone additional critical appraisal. The Cochrane Library contains systematic reviews that have been conducted in accordance with strict guidelines, but if the information you are looking for is not available in the Cochrane Library, then you will need to search other databases, such as MEDLINE, EMBASE, CINAHL and PsycInfo. The papers indexed in these databases are not appraised by the indexers, and consequently their quality is variable. This section contains some resources for appraising documents.

Critical appraisal means being able to look at a paper in an objective and structured way, so that you can be confident about the validity and quality of the paper.

If you are supporting a treatment decision based on a published paper, you want to be sure that the research has been carried out reliably and accurately without bias. Published papers are not always reliable and may not always be relevant to your patient population. The critical appraisal process should entail a fair assessment of the research, weighing up the strengths against weaknesses, and benefits against limitations.

The purpose of critical appraisal is to answer the following three questions:

1. What are the results?
2. Are the results valid?
3. How will these results help me in my work?

There are many checklists and tools available to help support critical appraisal, and some are listed below:

- Centre for Evidence-Based Medicine – checklists and tools
  www.cebm.net
- Critical Appraisal Skills Programme (CASP) – tools
  www.phru.nhs.uk/Pages/PHD/resources.htm
- School of Health and Related Research – online course
  www.shef.ac.uk/scharr/ir/units/critapp/
- Scottish Intercollegiate Guidelines Network – checklists
  www.sign.ac.uk/methodology/checklists.html

- What is critical appraisal?
  www.jr2.ox.ac.uk/bandolier/painres/download/whatis/What_is_
  criticalappraisal.pdf

Many institutions provide training in critical appraisal because it plays such an important role in evidence-based practice, so it is worth contacting your local librarian to see if your institution runs courses.

13. Further reading by topic or PubMed ID

This section lists articles that cover a range of topics featured in this book.

Critical appraisal

Jackson R, Ameratung S, Broad J, Connor J et al. The GATE frame: critical appraisal with pictures. ACP Journal Club 2006;144(2):A8–A11 (www.health.auckland.ac.nz/population-health/epidemiology-biostats/epiq/GATE%20in%20ACP.pdf).

Greenhalgh T (Greenhalgh T) How to read a paper. Papers that report drug trials. BMJ 1997 Aug 23;315(7106):480–3. [Review; no abstract available.] PMID: 9284672.

PMID: an easy way to search for papers is to remember the PubMed ID (PMID). So to search for the paper above, just enter the PMID number 9284672 in the search box.

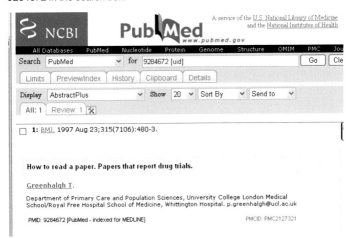

Evidence-based practice

Dawes M, Summerskill W, Glasziou P et al. Sicily statement on evidence-based practice. BMC Medical Education 2005;5:1 (www.biomedcentral. com/content/pdf/1472-6920-5-1.pdf).

Glasziou P, Haynes B. The paths from research to improved health outcomes. ACP Journal Club 2005 Mar-Apr;142(2):A8–10. [No abstract available.] PMID: 15739973

Filters

Kastner M, Wilczynski NL, Walker-Dilks C et al. Age-specific search strategies for Medline. Journal of Medical Internet Research 2006;8:4 (www.pubmedcentral.nih.gov/articlerender.fcgi?tool=pmcentrez&artid=17 94003).

Motschall E, Antes G, Klar R et al. Efficient Medline search filters for clinical queries. Conference: European Association for Health Information and Libraries (www.zbmed.de/fileadmin/pdf_dateien/EAHIL_2002/ motschall-proc.pdf).

Sampson M, Zhang L, Morrison A et al. An alternative to the hand searching gold standard: validating methodological search filters using relative recall. BMC Medical Research Methodology 2006;6:33 (www.pubmedcentral.nih. gov/picrender.fcgi?artid=1557524&blobtype=pdf)

Sandars S, Del Mar C. Clever searching for evidence: new search filters can help to find the needle in the haystack. British Medical Journal 2005;330(7501):1162–1163 (www.bmj.com/cgi/content/ full/330/7501/1162).

Formulating clinical questions

Huang X, Lin J, Demner-Fushman D. PICO as a knowledge representation for clinical questions. National Library of Medicine 2006 (http://mdot.nlm. nih.gov/pubs/ceb2006/pico-amia2006.pdf).

Richardson WS, Wilson MC, Nishikawa J, Hayward RSA. The well-built clinical question: a key to evidence-based decisions. ACP Journal Club 1995 Nov/Dec;A12–A13 (http://www.mclibrary.duke.edu/subject/ebm/ebm/ richardson.pdf)

Schardt C, Adams MB, Owens T, Keitz S, Fontelo P. Utilization of the PICO framework to improve searching PubMed for clinical questions. BMC Medical Informatics and Decision-Making 2007;7:16 (http://www.pubmedcentral.nih.gov/picrender.fcgi?tool=pmcentrez&artid=1904193&blobtype=pdf).

Publication types

Crumley ET, Wiebe N, Cramer K et al. Which resources should be used to identify RCT/CCTs for systematic reviews: a systematic review. BMC Medical Research Methodology 2005;5:24 (hwww.pubmedcentral.nih.gov/picrender.fcgi?tool=pmcentrez&artid=1232852&blobtype=pdf)

Fraser C, Murray A, Burr J. Identifying observational studies of surgical interventions in MEDLINE and EMBASE. BMC Medical Research Methodology 2006;6:41 (www.pubmedcentral.nih.gov/picrender.fcgi?tool=pmcentrez&artid=1569861&blobtype=pdf).

Golder S, McIntosh HM, Loke Y. Identifying systematic reviews of the adverse effects of healthcare interventions. BMC Medical Research Methodology 2006;6:22 (www.pubmedcentral.nih.gov/picrender.fcgi?tool=pmcentrez&artid=1481562&blobtype=pdf).

Haase A, Follmann M, Skipka G, Kirchner H. Developing search strategies for clinical practice guidelines in SUMSearch and Google Scholar and assessing their retrieval performance. BMC Medical Research Methodology 2007;7:28 (www.pubmedcentral.nih.gov/picrender.fcgi?tool=pmcentrez&artid=1925105&blobtype=pdf).

Haynes RB, Kastner M, Wilczynski NL et al . Developing optimal search strategies for detecting clinically sound and relevant causation studies in EMBASE. BMC Medical Informatics and Decision-Making 2005;5:8 (http://www.pubmedcentral.nih.gov/picrender.fcgi?tool=pmcentrez&artid=1087487&blobtype=pdf).

14. Glossary of terms

Abstract

This is a short, often word-limited to about 100–150 words, structured or unstructured summary of the paper. The abstract appears in healthcare databases and at the start of a published paper.

Adjacent (Adj)

This is also referred to as 'with'. It is useful when searching for phrases that contain smaller connecting words such as of, the, by, for, etc. For example, 'community with1 practice' will find results containing the phrase 'community of practice'.

Aggregator

Also known as a feed reader or a news reader, this is an online service that is used for collecting RSS feeds (see below). Many web browsers have a facility to collect RSS feeds. Alternatively, a service called Bloglines (www.bloglines.com/) is available.

And

This is a Boolean operator that narrows the search results so that all terms are searched for; e.g. 'venous thrombosis and compression stockings'.

Blog

This is an example of web 2.0 technology, and is short for Web log. It is an online journal where people can post news, comments and thoughts. Many resources, including journals, use blogs to promote new content. Blogger (www.blogger.com) and WordPress (http://wordpress.com) are examples of blog software.

Boolean operators

Boolean operators are words that facilitate the combination of search terms, allowing the search to be limited or widened.

Broader term

This is the opposite of narrowing a search and it means that the search is less specific regarding the search term, thus avoiding the issue of missing out on relevant research.

Browser

This is the software that lets you view the Internet/World Wide Web. Internet Explorer and Mozilla Firefox are both types of browser.

Citation

This provides all the information that is needed to find the research paper when the full text is not available online. A citation is made up of:

- Title of the paper
- Author(s)
- Source (e.g. journal title, date, volume, part/issue number, page numbers)

Citation index

This is a bibliographic tool that helps to track when and where a piece of research has been cited in subsequent pieces of research.

Citation manager

This is a piece of software that stores citations and abstracts retrieved from the search database. The stored items can then be manipulated and used in a format to support document creation, collation of references, etc. Examples of citation managers include:

- Reference Manager: www.refman.com
- EndNote: www.endnote.com/
- ProCite: www.procite.com/

Citation pearl searching

This is another method of searching for literature. It looks at:

- other papers by the same author(s);
- the references that the authors have used to see what papers those authors looked at;
- the keywords that the authors have used in their search strategy;
- related similar items – this option is appearing more often on databases.

Clinical Queries

This is a service that was originally developed by PubMed, which built filters into the database based on those created by the team at McMaster University. There are two types of filtered search available:

1. Question type – this search finds citations that correspond to a specific clinical study category, e.g. aetiology, diagnosis, therapy, prognosis or clinical prediction guides. There is also the option to create a narrow, specific search or a broad, sensitive search.
2. Systematic reviews – this search finds citations for systematic reviews, meta-analyses, reviews of clinical trials, evidence-based medicine, consensus development conferences and guidelines.

PubMed Clinical Queries is available at: www.ncbi.nlm.nih.gov/entrez/query/static/clinical.shtml

Combining

This activity helps to build an effective search strategy because it joins the terms together, using Boolean operators, so that relevant results are retrieved.

Controlled vocabulary

This is also known as Medical Subject Headings (MeSH), index terms or keywords; for any particular article, these comprise a few words that identify the content of the research and are added to the thesaurus or index.

Database

This is a searchable computer system that stores and indexes all the abstracts from the research. Examples include PubMed, CINAHL, PsycInfo, EMBASE and MEDLINE.

Descriptors

These are also known as controlled vocabulary, Medical Subject Headings (MeSH), index terms or keywords; for any particular article, they comprise a few words that identify the content of the research and are added to the thesaurus or index.

Email alerts

Many resources provide a service that lets users know when new content has been added or new articles have been published. The results are sent via email.

Explode term

This concept is part of the thesaurus feature, and enables the search to be extended to include narrower terms.

Feed reader

Also known as an aggregator or a news reader, this is an online service that is used for collecting RSS feeds (see below). Many web browsers have a facility to collect RSS feeds. Alternatively, a service called Bloglines (www.bloglines.com/) is available.

Filter

McMaster University have developed a set of search strategies that direct the database to find research of a particular publication type. By applying one of these filters, for example the filter for systematic reviews, to a search, the database will find all systematic reviews that match the search terms entered. PubMed was the first to offer this feature in the form of 'Clinical Queries', but now many other databases are incorporating filters.

Focus

This feature means that the database will search for the term as a major subheading, e.g. any records found will have the term describing an important aspect of the article.

Free text

The words are typed into the database as they would be spoken or spelled.

History

This feature appears on most databases and is a record of all the searches carried out during a particular search session.

Hyperlinks

These are electronic connections that take you to another page or somewhere else in the document.

Index terms

Also known as controlled vocabulary, Medical Subject Headings (MeSH) or keywords; for any particular article, they comprise a few words that identify the content of the research and are added to the thesaurus or index.

Information

This is facts, knowledge or concepts that have been received or communicated.

Internet

This is also known as the World Wide Web, and is a vast collection of knowledge and information on all topics, created by a range of authors, both expert and non-expert.

Keywords

These are also known as controlled vocabulary, Medical Subject Headings (MeSH), descriptors and index terms; for any particular article, they comprise a few words that identify the content of the research and are added to the thesaurus or index.

Knowledge

This is acquired on an individual basis, as a result of interaction and learning. It is also known as wisdom, expertise, tacit, intuition, etc.

Level of evidence

This is a hierarchy of study designs arranged according to their internal validity, or degree to which they are not susceptible to bias. They are available at: www.cebm.net/index.aspx?o=1025.

Limit

Databases have varying limit options. Some have very comprehensive options, for example MEDLINE, which allows the age to be broken up into 13 stages of life, including newborn, middle-aged, and aged. Limit options include language, publication type, gender, etc.

MeSH

This stands for Medical Subject Headings. It is a thesaurus of medical terms used by many databases and libraries to index and classify medical information. MeSH helps to overcome the issues of US/UK English and different terminology applied to identical concepts. MeSH is also known as controlled vocabulary or keywords.

Narrower term

This is a word that is much more specific, allowing the search to be more focused. For example, rather than searching for 'nurse' a narrower term might be 'community nurse'.

Natural language

The words are typed into the database as they would be spoken, without being refined.

Near

This is used as a Boolean operator and it means that all the words will be searched in a specific order, e.g. as a phrase.

News reader

Also known as an aggregator or feed reader, this is an online service that is used for collecting RSS feeds (see below). Many web browsers have a facility to collect RSS feeds. Alternatively, a service called Bloglines (www.bloglines.com/) is available.

Not

This is used as a Boolean operator and it means that only one of the terms will be searched for; e.g. 'contraception not oral' would exclude research on oral contraceptives.

Open access

This refers to research that is freely accessible to all via the World Wide Web. Biomed Central (www.biomedcentral.com/) is an example of a supplier of online open-access journals.

Open source

This refers to computer programs for which the source code has been made freely available by the authors so that it can be developed by other authors to create new programs. Linux (www.linux.org) is an example of the open-source initiative.

Or

This is used as a Boolean operator and it means that the database will search for one or other of the terms or for research containing both terms.

PICO

This is the acronym for a framework for building focused, clinical questions. The 'P' represents the patient or problem or population; the 'I' stands for intervention, e.g. the treatment; 'C' is for comparison, and is a stage that is not always necessary; and 'O' stands for outcome.

Primary research

This refers to original studies, such as a randomized controlled trial, cohort study, etc., where data are collected from experiments, observation and case studies.

Publication type

This describes the style of evidence; for example, it may be a research study, a letter responding to a published article, a report, a randomized controlled trial, a review, etc.

Respected authorities

These refer to societies, associations, royal colleges, etc. that inform and influence the development and activities of the professions they represent.

RSS feeds

This is web 2.0 software (see below) and is available on many sites. It is a method for notifying a subscriber of new content on websites or newly published research in journals. RSS feeds are recognizable by an orange button, either with XML, RSS or a symbol on it (as above). An aggregator/feed reader (see above) is required to collect the RSS feeds. A useful tutorial on RSS is available from Common Craft (commoncraft.com). The video called 'RSS in Plain English' is available here: www.commoncraft.com/rss_plain_english.

Search engines

Online tools to navigate the Internet, search for information, and retrieve relevant web pages. Examples include Alta Vista (http://www.av.com), Google (http://www.google.co.uk) and Yahoo (http://www.yahoo.co.uk).

Search strategy

A combination of carefully selected terms that, when entered into a database, will retrieve relevant papers to answer a focused clinical question, from which the terms originated.

Secondary research

An academic review of primary research studies to gain new insights on a specific topic (such as a systematic review).

Secondary sources

Secondary sources of information contain reviews of information originally published elsewhere. The Cochrane Library (www.theCochraneLibrary.com), the TRIP database (www.tripdatabase.com/) and evidence- based journals (http://clinicalevidence.bmj.com/ceweb/resources/useful_links.jsp) provide access to secondary research.

Sensitivity

This term applies to searching and statistics. In searching, it means that more relevant articles are retrieved, but at the expense of picking up more irrelevant results.

Single citation matcher

This is a service provided by PubMed that helps to locate the full reference of a research paper, when only partial information is available. Single citation manager is available at: www.ncbi.nlm.nih.gov/entrez/query/static/citmatch. html.

Social bookmarking

This is web 2.0 software (see below) and allows users to store bookmarks online so that they are accessible from any computer. The bookmarks can also be shared with colleagues, and can be catalogued or tagged by adding keywords. Connotea (www.connotea.org) and Del.icio.us (http://de.icio.us/) are examples of social bookmarking tools.

Source

This describes the location where the original research is published, e.g. book, journal, web address, etc.

Specificity

This term applies to searching and statistics. In searching, it means that it will retrieve mainly relevant results, but not all, thereby missing some key papers.

Subheadings

Subheadings appear as an option in the Advanced Search feature of most healthcare databases. They allow you to refine your search even further, by selecting one or more from a range of choices.

Summary

This is a shortened version of a document, e.g. a synopsis, providing the key points.

Synonyms

These are alternative terms meaning the same thing, e.g. venous thrombosis, deep vein thrombosis, etc.

Text word

Healthcare databases search for text words in the title or abstract of the document.

Thesaurus

This is also known as controlled vocabulary, Medical Subject Headings (MeSH) or keywords; for any particular article, they comprise a few words that identify the content of the research and are added to the thesaurus or index.

Uniform Resource Locators (URLs)

This is the address of a website, most commonly starting with 'http' (hyper text transfer protocol).

Web 2.0

This is the second generation of the Internet and provides tools that enable people to keep up to date with information, share knowledge and work together. Examples of web 2.0 technology include RSS, blogs, social bookmarking and wikis.

Wildcard

A wildcard is when a question mark is used in place of a letter when it is not clear whether the spelling is British English or American English or whether the term is singular or plural. For example, 'behavio?r' or 'wom?n'.

Wikis

Wikis are online spaces where groups of people can edit documents together. They are useful for people working on the same project but who are geographically spread. An example of wiki software is Wikispaces (http://www.wikispaces.com).

World Wide Web (WWW)

The World Wide Web, also known as the Internet, is a collection of knowledge and information on all topics, created by a range of authors both expert and non-expert.

Appendix I: Ten tips for effective searching

1. Turn the clinical problem into a question and pull out the keywords. The **PICO** (Patient/Problem, Intervention, Comparison, Outcomes) format is a good template to use because it enables you to be clear in the outcomes. Make a list of alternative terms that might be used for each of the major concepts – **never rely on any one term because you may miss out on relevant research!** For example, searching for the term 'mobile phones' will miss out many relevant articles, if you do not also search for 'cell phone' or 'cellular'.

2. When searching databases, start with a subject search and combine with a keyword search, for best results. Begin with a free-text search, entering and then combining most likely terms. Use truncation and wildcards to broaden your search:
   - use * or $ (depending on the database) to truncate words: e.g. nurs* will look for nurse, nurses, nursing;
   - use wildcard ? for alternative spellings: e.g. behavio?r will look for behaviour or behavior.

3. Find additional or related search terms from retrieved records:
   - abstracts/titles: free text terms;
   - MeSH fields: MeSH (i.e. thesaurus/subject) headings.

4. Focus your search using **Thesaurus** (also known as MeSH – Medical Subject Headings or Subject).

5. Combine search terms (free text or thesaurus) using Boolean operators:

AND	*all the search terms must appear in each record found*
OR	*at least one of the search terms must appear in each record found*
NOT	*the specified term must not appear in any of the results*

6. If **too many** records are retrieved, go back over the strategy and **narrow** the search:
   - use more specific or most relevant terms in free text;
   - use thesaurus search rather than free text;
   - use more specific or relevant MeSH terms;
   - select specific subheadings with MeSH terms;
   - add terms for other aspects of question (e.g. age or gender of patient), using AND;
   - use limit features (see tip 8 below).

7. If **too few** records are retrieved, go back over the strategy and **widen** the search:
   - use more terms: synonyms, related terms, broader terms (thesaurus or free text);
   - add in terms of related meaning with OR;
   - combine results of thesaurus and free-text searches;
   - use Explode feature of thesaurus, which will include narrower terms;
   - select All Subheadings with MeSH terms.

8. Limit search results at END of search by:
   - language of article;
   - checktags (human, animal, male, female);
   - publication type: e.g. RCTs, meta-analysis, reviews.

9. Review your search strategy on a regular basis and set up an alert so that you are kept up to date with new research.

10. Contact your local health librarian for more advice or make use of the help pages on your chosen information source.

Appendix 2: Teaching tips

This section includes some ideas for teaching the concepts of search skills to health professionals:

Imagine you are looking for a new car – icebreaker

At the start of a search skills session, show a picture of something you might want to buy, such as a car, and say: 'Imagine you are looking for a car; where would you look for choices?' Ask participants to shout out some ideas and write them on a flip chart. Answers might be: yellow pages, friends, adverts, critic reviews, surfing the Internet, television programmes, etc. Explain that you would use the same principles for finding the answers to clinical questions, for example asking colleagues, reading books and articles, surfing the Internet, databases, etc.

Name that database

There are many databases that cover health-related topics, and the number can be quite confusing. This exercise gives the participants a list of the databases available, together with a brief description, including details of content and period of cover. Divide the participants into groups and give them a list of scenarios or clinical questions. Ask them to work within their groups to choose the most suitable database(s) for answering the scenarios or clinical questions. This can also be used to identify which database is most suitable for different types of question, such as prognosis, therapy or diagnosis. The scenarios can then be used in the hands-on search session. Some examples of questions include:

1. You want to find out about the benefits of modern matrons (DH-Data, CINAHL).
2. You want to find out whether newborns should be vaccinated against chicken pox, if the mother has been exposed to the illness (MEDLINE/PubMed, EMBASE, CINAHL).
3. You want to find out articles about the effects of Prozac on someone suffering from depression (EMBASE, MEDLINE/PubMed).
4. You want to find out if psychological debriefing alleviates the symptoms of post-traumatic stress disorder (PsycInfo, EMBASE, MEDLINE/PubMed).
5. You want to find out if alternative therapies can help manage obesity (AMED, MEDLINE/PubMed).

Terminology mix and match

The aim of the glossary exercise is to familiarize people with the terminology used in searching, critical appraisal and research. You prepare one set of cards with the terms on them and another set with the definitions. You mix them all up, and the participants have to work together to match the pairs. You can have more than one set of cards depending on how big the group is. It is a useful exercise because it does provoke discussion and helps people to remember what the terms mean. Terms will differ depending on what is being taught.

Examples of cards:

Systematic review	A review of a clearly formulated question that uses systematic and explicit methods to identify, select and critically appraise relevant research, and to collect and analyse data from the studies that are included in the review.
Text word	Free-text fields refer to those words that have not been individually indexed in the database.
Thesaurus	Many databases include a list of controlled vocabulary used to standardize the indexing in the database. This enables the searcher to select and search for synonyms, related terms and preferred terms, and also to see descriptions of the terms.
Truncation	This symbol (often * or $) can be used when searching. The symbol acts as a substitute for any string of zero or more characters at the end of a word. For example, the search aggress* retrieves aggression, aggressive, aggressor. This symbol can be used anywhere in the search term, except as the first character.
Qualitative research	Research that uses words and aims to identify concepts and common themes. The research is based on opinions and statements, as opposed to statistics.
Quantitative research	Research in which the data are numerical and that seeks to test hypotheses by statistical analysis of the data.

Create more cards from the Glossary in this book.

Comparing different sources of information

An effective icebreaker for larger groups is to split them up and allocate three types of information source to each group: for example, Medline, colleagues and books for one group, and the Cochrane Library, the Internet and journals for the second group. An example to give to the groups is 'newspapers'. Give them about 10 minutes to discuss and list, within their groups, the advantages and disadvantages of their elected information sources. After 10 minutes, ask each group to feed back to the group as a whole, inviting brief comments. This exercise helps people to understand why you need to think about which are the best sources of information for people to use when searching for quality health information. Answers might include:

Information source	Advantages	Disadvantages
Book	<ul><li>easy to access</li><li>greater depth of coverage than journals</li><li>overview of subject</li><li>portable</li><li>reduced cost – borrow from library</li><li>good reference</li></ul>	<ul><li>quickly out of date</li><li>quality of indexing varies</li><li>time consuming to search/scan</li><li>expensive</li><li>access to libraries may be limited</li><li>author/publisher bias</li></ul>

Etc.

Record your own favourite websites

Index

TRIP (Turning Research Into Practice) database 17–18